Diabetes 101:

A Patient Handbook

Sonia Talwar, M.D.

Editor

Syed Mohammed Rizvi, B.S.

With Contributions From

Sameer Verma, M.D.
Barbara Capozzi, D.O.
Abhinav K. Vulisha, M.B.B.S
Shilpa Malik, M.M.S.

Disclaimer

This book is not intended to replace a physician's advice. While medical professionals are writing this book, there is no substitute for personalized medical care. Every person has individual needs and not every statement in this book will apply to your personal health. You should consult your doctor before making any changes in your healthcare or following any advice you may find in this book.

Table of Contents

1 | What is Diabetes?

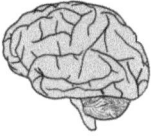

"Breath is the bridge which connects life to consciousness, which unites your body to your thoughts."

Thich Nhat Hanh (b. 1926)

Diabetes is an illness that once diagnosed is something that requires lifelong management and care. It is defined as increased levels of sugar in the blood. There may be many etiologies and concomitant factors causing increased sugar levels and an eventual diagnosis of Diabetes Mellitus. However, the two main principles surrounding the formation of diabetes is that the pancreas is not producing enough insulin, or the body has become resistant to the natural insulin that is being produced. This chapter outlines the basic anatomical principles pertaining to diabetes.

Pancreas - a glandular organ that is part of the digestive system and is also considered part of the endocrine system. It's an endocrine gland that produces insulin as well as other hormones and enzymes essential for digestion. The enzymes help to further break down the carbohydrates, proteins, and lipids.

Insulin - a hormone that is produced by beta (β) cells of the pancreas. It is essential to regulate sugar, carbohydrate and fat metabolism in the body. In addition it causes the liver, muscle cells, and fat tissue to absorb free sugar from the blood.

Glucagon - a hormone secreted by the pancreas that raises blood sugar levels. It works in conjunction with insulin to keep a homeostatic level of sugar. Glucagon causes the liver to convert stored glycogen into glucose.

Glycogen – a molecule that is made of many molecules of glucose. It acts as a form of stored energy. Glycogen is made and stored in the liver and the muscles. The glycogen that is stored in the muscles and cells are converted to glucose when the body needs a more efficient source of energy.

Liver – an organ of the digestive system that is involved in the body's detoxification, protein building and digestion. The liver also plays a major role in the body's metabolic function. It's role in diabetes revolves around glycogen storage and its role in changing sugar levels.

Type 1 Diabetes

Type 1 diabetes results from a loss of pancreatic beta cells. Usually this is due to autoimmune destruction of the β cells of the pancreas that produce the body's endogenous insulin. Due to the resulting lack of insulin blood sugars levels become elevated. The lack of insulin pricing cells leads to a increase in urine sugars as well. The classical symptoms of diabetes in general are polyuria (frequent urination), polydipsia (increased thirst), polyphagia (increased hunger), and weight loss.

Type 2 Diabetes

Type 2 diabetes is a metabolic disorder that is characterized by high blood glucose which is caused by development of resistance to the body's own insulin, decreased insulin production or a combination of both.

The most common symptoms associated with this type of diabetes are excess thirst, frequent urination, and constant hunger. Type 2 diabetes makes up the overwhelming majority of diabetes cases and is greatly associated with obesity as it is thought to be the major cause followed by diet and genetics.

Gestational Diabetes

Gestational diabetes is when women who have not been previously diagnosed with diabetes exhibit high blood sugar levels during pregnancy. It is thought that the cause of gestational diabetes is when the insulin receptors do not function properly due to the physiologic changes associated with pregnancy. It has been theorized that factors such as the presence of human placental lactogen interferes with insulin receptors which causes inappropriately elevated blood sugar levels. There are relatively few signs or symptoms except for elevated blood sugar levels.

Steroid Induced Diabetes

Steroid induced diabetes describes increased blood sugars levels that are caused by glucocorticoid steroid therapy which is being taken for another medical condition. This drug induced diabetes is usually temporary in nature as long as the steroids are being taken. Symptoms tend to be minimal as this is a transient condition.

Latent Autoimmune Diabetes (LADA)

Latent autoimmune diabetes is considered a slow-onset type 1 autoimmune diabetes which occurs in adults. It is possible that up to half of all adult patients with non-obesity related diabetes may have this type of diabetes.

Maturity Onset Diabetes of the Young (MODY)

Maturity onset diabetes of the young is a term used to refer to many types of diabetes that are genetic in nature which lead to a disruption insulin production. This type of diabetes is often seen in a younger population but should not be confused with Type 1 or Type 2 diabetes mellitus.

Metabolic Syndrome

Metabolic syndrome is a condition defined as a cluster of three or more of the following risk factors in adults which include increased abdominal circumference, hypertension, elevated cholesterols, and elevated blood sugars. Metabolic syndrome is considered to be a pre-diabetic condition and should be treated aggressively to prevent formation of diabetes.

"

**Diabetes...
It's pronounced
(di-a-bea-teez),
& NOT
(die-ah-BEAT-us)
Because we refuse
to let it BEAT US.**

"

2 | Symtomatology

"I claim that in losing the spinning wheel we lost our left lung. We are, therefore, suffering from galloping consumption. The restoration of the wheel arrests the progress of the fell disease."

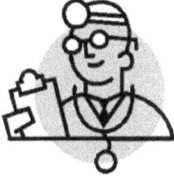

Mahatma Gandhi (1869-1948)

Increased sugar levels in the blood may manifest as many different signs and symptoms. In this chapter we plan to outline some of the most commonly seen and why they occur. Symptomatology of diabetes is similar in both Type 1 and Type 2.

Symptoms

Polyuria

Polyuria is an increased frequency of urination that is present in both types of diabetes; however it is greater in Type 1. Increased urination occurs due forced filtration of the blood (osmotic dieresis) which is secondary to persistently elevated sugar levels. This phenomenon is the body's way of ridding the extra sugar as well as free water and electrolytes. Bedwetting or nocturnal enuresis may be the first sign of DM in children.

Polydipsia

Polydipsia or excessive thirst is caused by the polyuria that is often seen in diabetes. It is a result of the hyperosmolar state that is caused by increased sugar levels. As mentioned above increased sugar levels lead to increased urination which in turn leads to dehydration. This dehydration leads to increased thirst and increased water intake.

Weakness and Fatigue

Weakness, fatigue and weight loss despite normal or increased appetite is a common feature seen in diabetes, with an affinity for type 1. In type one this weight loss will occur over a short period of time which it is initially due to increased water loss. Weight loss seen in diabetes takes place over time unintentionally. This loss of weight is primarily due to reduced muscle mass.

Paresthesia

Parathesia is a feeling of tingling, prickling, or burning of a person's skin. It may be present in type 1 DM but is more commonly seen in Type 2 due to the chronicity of disease. The sensation is caused by damage of the peripheral sensory nerves. With regulation of sugar levels it has been reported to improve.

Signs

Obesity

Obesity, now considered a disease, is which excess body fat has accumulated to the extent that it may have detrimental effects on your body. Obesity is often associated with formation of insulin resistance, a major component of diabetes.

Acanthosis nigricans (skin lesion)

Acanthosis nigricans is a velvety darkening of the skin. It is often associated with insulin resistance and is seen mainly in Type 2 DM. It is usually found in body folds such as the back and side folds of the neck the armpits, the groin, and other areas.

Increased Infections

The presence of excess sugar in the blood may cause an increase in candidal vaginitis (yeast infections) with a reddened, inflamed vulvar area and a profuse whitish discharge in women. Men who get infection of the genitalia have reddish appearance of the penis and/or prepuce with eroded white papules and a white discharge. Some patients may also experience oral infections.

Impaired wound healing

Patients who maintain elevated plasma glucose levels are prone to infections as mentioned above. One of the causes of this increase is impaired wound healing which is caused by destruction of the micro-vessels.

> *By 2050 it is thought that approximately 100 million Americans, one third of the population will be diabetic, 90% of who will not be diagnosed.*

"

I'm STRONGER
Than
Diabetes.

"

3 | Diagnosing Your Disease

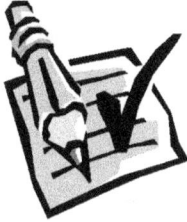

"Natural forces within us are the true healers of disease."

Hippocrates (460 BC – 377 BC)

The prominent feature of diabetes is increased blood sugar levels. On this basis the diagnosis of diabetes mellitus is centered on fasting blood glucose levels as well as how the body reacts to ingestion of a measured amount of sugar. In this chapter we plan to outline the testing and diagnostics that go into making a diagnosis of diabetes.

Fasting Glucose

A fasting glucose test or fasting blood sugar is measured via a blood sample that is taken 8, 12 or 14 hours after eating and fasting (Table). This test can be done at a lab that exclusively does blood work or at your physicians' office/home using a glucometer. A fasting sugar level of 100 mg/dL (5.6 mmol/L) to 125 mg/dL (6.9 mmol/L) is associated with an increased risk for diabetes (impaired glucose tolerance).

Oral Glucose Tolerance Test (OGTT)

This is a test that was widely used to diagnose diabetes but now with the ease of blood work it is not used as much anymore. In preparation for the test a patient is instructed to fast for an 8-12 hour period. The test begins with a baseline blood sample that is drawn to measure fasting sugar. The patient is then given a measured dose of glucose solution to drink. Blood is drawn in intervals at 1 hour and 2 hours. Results will be interpreted by your physician.

Postprandial Glucose Test

A postprandial glucose test determines the amount of sugar in the blood after a meal (Table). In healthy people blood sugar levels increase slightly after eating. Food consumption leads to increased sugars in the blood which is regulated by the pancreas. Diabetic patients have a reduced ability to counter the increasing sugars levels which causes hyperglycemia. A normal postprandial glucose 2 hours after eating a meal is considered to be <140 mg/dL. Diabetic patients usually have levels > 200 mg/dL.

Glycated Hemoglobin (HemoglobinA1c)

The hemoglobin A1c is a quantitative measure of how many of your red blood cells have a sugar molecule attached to the hemoglobin molecule inside of them. (Table) The normal percent of glycated hemoglobin in the body is roughly between 4-6%. This test may be done at a laboratory or may be performed in some specialized offices. The lifespan of a red blood cell is approximately 120 days. The HemoglobinA1c measurement reports about glucose control over the previous 8-12 weeks.

Table 1: Diagnosis Criteria for Diabetes

Criteria for the Diagnosis of Diabetes			
	Normal Glucose Tolerance	Impaired Glucose Tolerance (Prediabetes)	Diabetes Mellitus
Fasting Plasma Glucose (mg/dl)	<100	100-125 (impaired fasting glucose)	> 126
2 hour oral glucose tolerance test (mg/dl)	<140	≥140-199 (impaired glucose tolerance)	≥ 200
HbA1C (%)	<5.7	5.7-6.4	≥6.5
Symptoms and random glucose level (mg/dL)	-------	------	≥200

Your A1c Goal

In most labs, the normal range is 4-5.9 % and in poorly controlled diabetes, its 8.0% or above. The American Diabetes Association currently recommends an A1c goal of less than 7.0%, while other groups such as the American Association of Clinical Endocrinologists recommend a goal of less than 6.5%.

While A1c test result can be reported as a percentage, it can also be reported as a number, called estimated Average glucose or eAG. In general an aAG of 154mg/dl is the goal for most people with diabetes.

A1C%	eAG mg/dl
5	97
6	126
7	154
8	183
9	212
10	240
11	269

Other Tests Your Doctor May Order

Spirometry

Spirometry is a routinely performed breathing test that assesses how well your lungs function. During this test, you will be asked to blow into a tube which is connected to a machine. This machine, or a spirometer, measures how much air your lungs can hold (forced vital capacity or FVC) and how fast you can blow air out (forced expiratory volume in one second or FEV_1). Along with a doctor's examination, spirometry can help determine how severe your COPD is. Values are expressed as percentage (%) of predicted. Predicted values are determined from your age, sex and height.

Pulmonary Function Testing (PFTs)

Pulmonary function testing is a commonly used test, ordered by the physician to evaluate the function of lungs. This testing involves the use of machinery to perform breathing tests to measure the size of lungs, the state of the airways of the lungs and the ability of the lungs to exchange oxygen and carbon dioxide.

Patients are asked to withhold long acting lung medications for 12 hours and short acting lung medications for 4 hours prior to testing. Patients are asked not to engage in vigorous physical exercise at least 4 hours prior to testing. Patients may be asked for a sample of blood to be drawn to measure the amount of the oxygen and carbon dioxide in the blood. This can be done by a certified Respiratory Therapist using a local anesthetic called lidocaine to numb the area over the artery in which the needle is inserted. Patients may be asked to inhale medication to open the airways in the lungs. This allows the doctors to determine how well the lungs respond to the type of medication.

6 Minute Walk Test (6MWT)

A 6MWT is a test used to find out how much you are able to exercise. The test will measure how far you can walk on a flat surface in 6 minutes. This test will allow your physician or respiratory therapist to determine your exercise capacity.

Cardio-Pulmonary Exercise Test

Another very important method for assessing prognosis in advanced lung disease is cardiopulmonary exercise testing (CPET). CPET involves measurement of oxygen consumption and carbon dioxide exhalation during exercise. Based on the results of this test and measurements of oxygen consumption your physician can better gauge how your disease is progressing and how to further manage your advanced lung disease.

Methacholine Challenge Test

Methacholine is a drug that causes narrowing of the airways. The degree of narrowing can be quantified by performing a spirometry. People with a history of hyperreactive airways such as asthmatics, will react to lower doses of drug. In addition to assessing the reversibility of a particular condition, a medication (bronchodilator) is administered to counteract the effects of the methacholine before repeating the spirometry tests. This is commonly referred to as a reversibility test and may help in distinguishing asthma from chronic obstructive pulmonary disease.

Bronchoscopy

Bronchoscopy is a common diagnostic procedure, usually done in an outpatient setting that allows your doctor to look inside your lungs and is routinely used for biopsies of shadows or changes on x-rays or CT scans. The bronchoscope is a thin, flexible tube with a tiny camera on the end and is inserted through the nose or mouth into the lungs. Bronchoscopy is a safe diagnostic procedure and carries little risk.

Abdominal Aortic Aneurysm ultrasound

A test that measures the size of the major artery that is located in the stomach area. This test is recommended 1 times only for men aged 65-75 years who have ever smoked.

Angiogram or Arteriogram

In an angiogram or arteriogram, dye is injected into the blood vessels using a catheter (small tube) and X-rays are taken. This test shows whether arteries are narrowed or blocked. A coronary angiogram checks for narrowing or blockages in the blood vessels that go to the heart. A cerebral arteriogram checks the blood vessels that go to the brain.

Angioplasty

Angioplasty, also called balloon angioplasty, is a procedure used to remove a blockage in a blood vessel to the heart (coronary angioplasty) or the brain. A small tube with a balloon attached is threaded into the narrowed or blocked blood vessel. Then the balloon is inflated, opening the narrowed artery. A wire tube, called a stent, may be left in place to help keep the artery open.

Ankle Brachial Index

A test called an ankle brachial index or ABI is used to diagnose peripheral artery disease (PAD). The health care provider compares the blood pressure in the ankle with that in the arm. Lower blood pressure in the lower part of the leg compared with the pressure in the arm may indicate PAD.

Cardiac catheterization

Left heart cardiac catheterization is used in conjunction with other tests. A small tube is inserted into an artery and guided into the blood vessel of the heart. It helps to locate blockages in the heart vessels and allows your cardiologist to perform an on the spot angioplasty.

Right Heart Catheterization

Here, a small tube is passed in the right side of the heart to measure the pressures in the pulmonary artery. This is the gold standard test for diagnosing pulmonary artery hypertension.

Chest X Ray

A chest X-ray shows the size and shape of the heart and can also show congestion in the lungs.

Coronary Artery Bypass Graft (CABG)

During a coronary artery bypass graft, also called a bypass or CABG (pronounced "cabbage"), a blood vessel taken from the leg, wrist, or chest is attached to the coronary artery to bypass a blockage and restore blood flow to the heart. A bypass graft can also be used for blood vessels leading to the brain.

CT Scan

A CT (computed tomography), also called a CAT scan, uses special scanning techniques to provide images of the lungs. You may be given a contrast prior to the test then this study is called as CT Angiography. This test allows your physician to evaluate your pulmonary arteries to look for any clots in them.

Dual X-ray Absorptiometry (DEXA)

DEXA was developed to screen for compromised bone health in the elderly. DEXA uses low dose radiation to measure bone density in the spine, hip, and whole body. DEXA measures "density" of bone but does not indicate the quality of bone. DEXA results are presented as standard deviation scores. According to the World Health Organization, osteoporosis is defined as bone mineral density standard deviation score (BMD-T) < 2.5; a bone density in this low range predicts future fracture risk. In children and adolescents, the use of a BMD-T is inappropriate and a BMD-Z must be used. How well BMD-Z predicts fracture risk in younger individuals is less well established. Thus, osteoporosis is defined in children and younger adults as BMD-Z<-2 and a history of significant fractures, including long bone fractures of the upper and lower extremities and compression fractures of the spine. For those on steroid therapy, such as prednisone, it is important to have a DEXA scan on a yearly basis.

Echocardiogram

An echocardiogram uses high-frequency sound waves (ultrasound) to produce images of the heart and blood vessels. Results indicate whether the heart is pumping blood correctly. It also allows us to estimate the pressure in the pulmonary arteries. This is good screening test when your health care provider wants to rule out pulmonary artery hypertension. A stress echocardiogram uses either exercise or medication and ultrasound to provide images of the heart and blood vessels under stress.

Electrocardiogram (EKG, ECG)

An electrocardiogram, also called an ECG or EKG, provides information on heart rate and rhythm and shows whether there has been any damage or injury to the heart muscle.

Exercise Perfusion Test (Nuclear Cardiac Stress Test)

An exercise perfusion test, also called a stress nuclear perfusion test, uses small amounts of radioactive material to produce images of blood flow to the heart as you exercise.

Exercise Stress Test

Exercise stress tests are used to find heart disease that is evident only during physical activity. It can also be used to help a patient choose the most appropriate physical activity program. Also called a treadmill test, a stress test uses an ECG to measure how the heart performs during activity, such as walking on a moving treadmill. A medication stress test uses medication instead of exercise to increase the heart rate.

Holter Monitoring

A Holter monitor is a small, portable machine that records the heart's electrical activity. The person wearing the monitor keeps track of symptoms and activities for the evaluation period. Readings on the machine are compared with the symptoms.

Magnetic Resonance Imaging (MRI)

MRI uses special scanning techniques to provide images of body tissues. MRA (magnetic resonance angiography) uses MRI to examine blood vessels.

Nerve Conduction Study (NCS)

A nerve conduction study is a diagnostic procedure that is routinely used to evaluate nerve function. This test is able to especially measure the ability of electrical conduction of both motor and sensory nerves.

Nuclear Ventriculography

Nuclear ventriculography also called radionuclide ventriculography uses small amounts of radioactive material to check heart function either while the body is at rest or during exercise. This test can also be used to check the blood vessels that go to the brain.

Ventilation Perfusion Scan

In this test, small amounts of radioactive material are injected in to the veins to evaluate the flow of blood through the lungs. This test is generally used to help diagnose presence of clots in the lungs, which is known as a pulmonary embolism.

Positron Emission Tomography (PET)

A PET scan uses special scanning techniques to provide images of body tissues. It helps to identify any tissue in the body that may be malignant (cancerous).

People with diagnosed diabetes have health care costs 2.3 times higher than what expenditures would be in the absence of diabetes.

"

Every human being is the author of their own disease.

"

4 | Diabetes Management

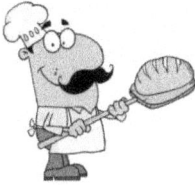

"The best doctor gives the least medicines."

Benjamin Franklin (1706-1790)

Since diabetes is a chronic condition, self management plays an important role in managing it. To successfully take care of your disease you must take an active part in maintaining your health. Meticulous monitoring of your blood sugar levels, diet, exercise, lifestyle modification, and patient education is essential to living with diabetes. This chapter will outline some strategies you can utilize to better maintain your health and change your lifestyle to help with your diabetes.

Nutrition and Diabetes

A healthy person should aim to get 45% to 65% of their calories from carbohydrates, with active individuals aiming for 55% to 65%. As for protein a healthy individual should aim to get about 10% to 35% of their calories. Fats are also essential to our well being, a healthy individual should aim to get 20% to 35% of their calories from fat.

Proteins

While protein can be used for energy when carbohydrates and fat are in short supply, protein's major role is building muscle, making blood and other body tissues. Many people consume meat products as a source of protein. It is important to know that red meats such as beef are linked to increased risk of heart disease. Good sources of protein include eggs, poultry (white meat), soy and whey.

Carbohydrates

Carbohydrates are the body's main source of energy. However, in diabetes they are the main culprit for increasing blood sugars and hemoglobinA1c. They may come in the form of simple sugars such as sucrose and fructose or in wheat products such as breads and pastas. While coping with diabetes you have to try to curb your cravings for carbohydrates. You will have to make adjustments and opt for whole wheat bread, whole wheat pastas and in some cases eliminate as many carbohydrates as possible.

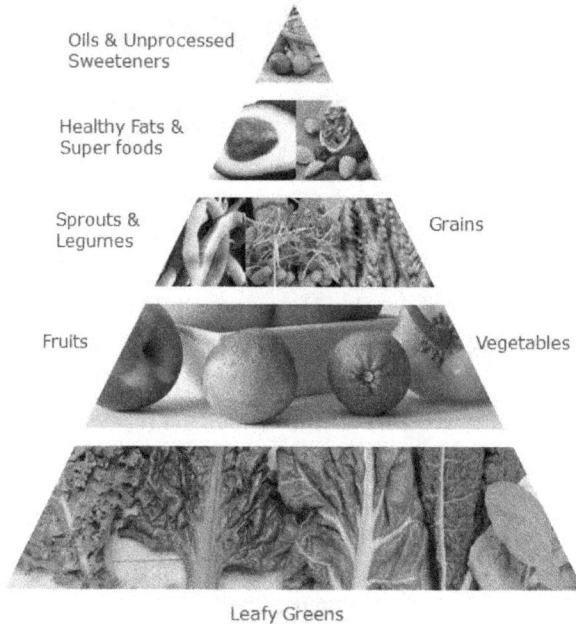

Oils & Unprocessed Sweeteners

Healthy Fats & Super foods

Sprouts & Legumes

Grains

Fruits

Vegetables

Leafy Greens

Fats

Fats are a common component of many foods. It is important to keep in mind that not all fats are bad and they might not be associated with cholesterol. Foods that are high in cholesterol and saturated fats come mostly from animal sources. To differentiate between saturated and unsaturated fats you can see how they act at certain temperatures. Saturated fats turn solid in cool temperatures, for example butter, or the layer of fat on top of a pot of chicken soup that's been in the refrigerator. Polyunsaturated fats do not contain cholesterol. These fats are from plant sources and they remain liquid at cold temperatures for example olive oil.

When you consume fat, make an effort to ensure that it is the polyunsaturated kind. Avoid animal fats such as butter, and cut down on fatty meats as these foods are high in cholesterol. Before you buy prepared products, read the labels. Many prepared foods list the cholesterol content on the ingredient panel. If you can buy either a product made with butter or one made with corn oil, choose the one made with corn oil.

More recently as a community we have become of aware of a different type of fat called trans-fats. Trans-fats are a type of unsaturated fat that have a different chemical configuration than typical saturated and unsaturated fats. These trans-fats are created by the processing and hydrogenation of unsaturated fats. These types of fats may be found naturally in the plant kingdom and in certain meat products like beef. Trans-fats have been associated with increased incidence of cardiac disease. They should be avoided whenever possible.

Table 8: Healthy vs. Less Healthy Fats

Healthy Fats	Less Healthy or Unhealthy Fats
Monounsaturated Fats • Olive oil • Peanut oil • Sesame oil • Variety of nut and seed oils: peanut, almond, macadamia nut, sesame • Avocados, olives • Full-fat ice cream	**Saturated Fats** • Butter • Lard • Tropical oils such as coconut, palm, palm kernel, cocoa butter • Fatty meats • Whole milk
Polyunsaturated Fats • Corn oil • Soybean oil • Sunflower oil • Safflower oil • Oil found in fish, salmon, tuna, mackerel, sardines, herring, anchovies	**Trans (Hydrogenated) Fats** • Shortening • Hard stick margarine (check labels) • Many baked goods, especially processed ones (check labels): croissants,

• Variety of nut and seed oils: walnut, pumpkin, flax • Heart-healthy spreads, such as Benecol and Take Control (if used two to three times a day in place of regular margarine or butter, these products may lower cholesterol by up to 14 percent	doughnuts, muffins, biscuits, chips, crackers, cookies, cakes • Fried foods, such as French fries, chicken nuggets, fish sticks

Lifestyle change Diet

Total fat	25-35% of total calories
Saturated fat*	< 7% of total calories
Carbohydrates	40-50% of total calories +
Fiber	20-30 gm/d
Protein	15-25% of total calories
Cholesterol	< 200 mg/d
Total calories	Sufficient to maintain desirable body weight

* Trans fats also raise LDL cholesterol and should be kept to a minimum

+ Most as complex carbohydrates from whole grains, fruits, vegetables

The Mediterranean Diet

Recently the Mediterranean diet has been shown to be beneficial for patients who are suffering from cardiovascular disease. This diet which is high in monounsaturated and omega-3 fatty acids can play an important role in the prevention of atherosclerotic disease. A study showed that patients who suffered from heart attack and adhered to a diet providing increased levels of alpha-linolenic acid (from olive oil and canola oil) or usual dietary instruction showed a 70% reduction in all-cause mortality.

Salt and Fluid Intake

United Stated Drug Administration (USDA) guidelines include recommendations for the general population. It has been recommended that no one should consume more than 2,300 milligrams of salt per day. Those who are age 51 and older and those who are African American or have high blood pressure, diabetes, or chronic kidney disease should consume no more than 1,500 milligrams per day.

As for fluid intake, the amount of fluid in your body is related to your consumption of fluid and particularly to your sodium intake. Sodium intake can greatly affect your fluid retention and may increase blood pressure and exacerbate heart and lung disease. Remember that some foods are full of liquid. For example, a cup of gelatin dessert has almost as much water as a cup of juice.

Hints to Reduce Salt/Sodium

Excessive salt/sodium intake may cause your body to retain fluid. This extra fluid volume often increases blood volume. It then becomes more difficult for your heart to circulate the blood. Breathing may become more difficult to keep up with the extra energy needs.

- Take the salt shaker off the table, only use during cooking.
- Flavor with herbs and spices, onions, garlic and pepper.
- Use fresh meats, fruits and vegetables. Processed foods are usually high in sodium.
- Read food labels and avoid products which use the words salt, sodium (Na), or soda in the first three ingredients.
- Consult your physician before using salt substitutes.

Here are some other suggestions to help you limit the amount of carbohydrate and increase your intake of good fats

- Eat enough calories to attain and maintain desired body weight.
- Eat fewer foods high in fat. These include: dairy and meat products, fried foods, oils, sauces, salad dressings, granola, party crackers and dips, fast foods, convenience foods and commercial pastries.
- Use artificial sweeteners.

- Eat a balanced diet and a variety of foods at each meal. "Balanced" means a protein source (meat or dairy product, beans or peas), carbohydrates (fruits, vegetables, grains and starches), fats (oil or margarine) and fluid at each meal.
- Substitute polyunsaturated fats for saturated fats whenever possible. Saturated fats are usually animal fats, found in dairy and meat products (such as butter, cream cheese, creamy salad dressings, visible and "hidden" meat fat, bacon, luncheon meats, sausage and hot dogs, fried foods), but sometimes are vegetable fats, as in chocolate, or coconut and palm oils. Polyunsaturated fats are only from vegetable sources: vegetable oils and margarine (especially tub margarines), nuts, avocados, olives and un-hydrogenated peanut butter. Eat more fish, poultry and veal in place of beef, lamb, pork and cheese. Use sunflower, corn, sunflower, soybean and cottonseed oils and margarines.
- Eat more complex carbohydrates and less refined, simple sugars. Complex carbohydrates are: fresh fruits and vegetables, whole-grained and enriched cereals (bread, cereals, rice, pasta, grits, oatmeal, cracked wheat and bran), potatoes, corn, peas, beans, lentils. Simple sugars are: sugar, honey, jam, jelly, sodas, candy, cookies, cake, processed foods and beverages, sugar-coated cereals. Eat complex carbohydrates for vitamins, minerals, energy, fiber, water and fewer calories.
- Use water-packed fruit or fruit with no added sugar.
- Use artificially sweetened jams, jellies and hard candies.
- If you have certain favorite foods you are not sure about, ask your dietitian if they are high in carbohydrate. Your dietitian may suggest ways that other foods can be used to balance the carbohydrate in those things you most enjoy.

Fiber

Fiber is a portion of vegetables, fruits, grains, and beans which passes through our digestive tract into the large intestine nearly completely undigested. Fiber aids bowel function, weight control, and may play a role in reducing cholesterol levels and carbohydrates absorption. Foods that are high in fiber include:

- Whole grain breads and cereals: bran, whole wheat, rye and pumpernickel

- Fresh fruits, fresh vegetables and salads
- Legumes: chick peas, lentils, beans, and peas

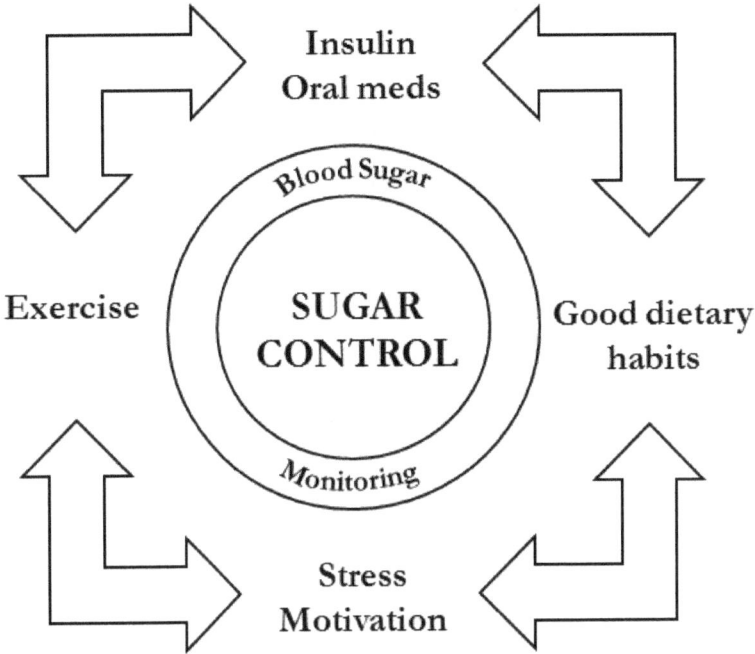

Beverages

Drinking 6-8 glasses of fluid a day helps to keep mucous thin and easier to cough up. Water, low calorie fruit juices, decaffeinated coffee or tea and milk are recommended beverages. Milk does not cause thickened saliva as many believe. Alcohol, fruit-flavored drinks, and soft drinks should be avoided since they are high in calories and contain little nutritional value.

Vitamin Supplements

Vitamin supplements are not necessary if you follow a well balanced diet. If you habitually eat a poor balanced diet you may benefit from a multi-vitamin. Consult your physician prior to beginning a new vitamin regimen.

"

**Managing your
Diabetes
Is not a science,
It is an Art.**

"

5 | Changing your habits

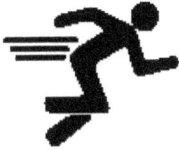

"Water, air and cleanness are the chief articles in my pharmacy."

Napoleon I (1769-1821)

A lot of your health maintenance is up to you. As you have you read the previous chapters you know that changing some habits to take better care of yourself may help your diabetes. Maybe you'd like to change some of your habits but you're stuck and you feel as though is very hard to start. Changing habits can be hard to do. But you can learn a step-by-step approach that will help you reach your goals. How can you start to change your habits? Every change a person makes in life involves several stages:

- Pre-contemplation - Maybe you think that a change would help but you're not ready or interested. You feel the change would be too hard to make.
- Contemplation - You're thinking about making a change, but not right away. At this stage, the costs of making the change still outweigh the benefits.
- Preparation - You're ready to make the change within the month. You've made a realistic plan and you've gathered what you need to carry out your plan.
- Action - You've taken action and started your new routine. But sometimes you're tempted to go back to your previous habits.
- Maintenance - After more than 6 months of your new routine, you're used to doing it. It's now a habit.

To change a habit, you have to realize what stage you are in. Once a person has established which stage he/she is in, the individual is more equipped and likely to act.

Ideal Body Weight

It is possible to eat your way to a great health. General guidelines you need to follow are: getting rid of junk food, and consuming sufficient protein (the USDA recommends 10-30 grams a day). The protein in diet should be from poultry or plant based protein saturated fat, high sodium food, prepackaged food.

Diet and Weight Management Pearls

- To limit the amount of food you consume in a sitting drink a full glass of water (8 ounces) immediately prior to eating. This water will take up some space in the stomach and stretch it triggering fullness centers in the brain. This will trick your mind into thinking that you do not need much more food to be full.
- Drink six to eight glasses of water a day. Proper hydration allows your body to shed any excess water that is stored in your fat cells. Not only will you lose your water weight but you body will function more efficiently.
- Start eating your meals out of smaller vessels. For example instead of having dinner in a full sized dinner plate start using a quarter plate. The purpose of this is to trick your mind into thinking that you have already had a sufficient portion. When going back for a second serving your mind will alert you that you are getting a second serving.
- Pre-cut vegetables into snack size portions. Place them in Ziploc sandwich back and keep them in the refrigerator front and center. This technique allows you to quickly open the fridge and get a snack that is healthy and delicious without much thinking. It also prevents you from eating some unhealthy snack like ice cream or chips and dip.
- Label the calories on all food with a big bold marker. Labeling all the items in your fridge with the calories will let you see how many calories you will get from a particular for before you grab it. The same goes for all pantry items and prepared foods.

What is a Serving?

While planning on how to count your calories and manage your portion sizes it is important to have an idea of what exactly a serving is. Most food items have nutritional information on them that is based on a serving. A serving may be different for different foods. Below you will find a table that tries to simplify what a serving should be..

Everyday household items can be used as guidelines for healthy serving sizes!

Household Item	Serving	Food
Deck of Cards	3-4 Ounces	Beef, Chicken, Pork, Salmon
Checkbook	~3 Ounces	Lean Fish Fillet
Compact Disk	~1 Ounce	Lean meat Pancake Waffle
Baseball	1 Cup	Cooked Pasta Cold Cereal Raw Vegetable
Tennis Ball	½ Cup	Cooked Vegetable Ice Cream Piece of Fruit

Golf Ball	~2 Tablespoons ~1/4 Cup	Peanut Butter Dried fruit, nuts
4 Dice	~1 Ounce	Cheese
Computer Mouse	1 Small	Potato
Your thumb	1 Tablespoon	Olive Oil Dressing Mayonnaise

Diet

The staple of diabetes management is management of diet. It is known that diets high in fats, sugar and starches in combination with low fiber have been linked to the development of diabetes. More recently, dietary studies have shown that vegetable oils and polyunsaturated fats have a role in lowering the chance for developing Type 2 diabetes. On the other hand, trans-fats, found in many fried foods, increase the chance of developing the disease.

Write down all blood glucose results in a log or record book. Bring them with you to all of your appointments. Your results will help you and your healthcare team will make decisions about your diabetes treatment plan. For a list of diabetes medications please refer to Appendix 4.

Keeping Track of Your Sugar

An important component of managing your diabetes is keeping track of your sugar by maintaining a finger stick diary. Finger sticking involves obtaining a small blood sample so you can check the blood sugar at that specific moment. This is something that used to be cumbersome but over the years has become something simple to do. Most people are familiar with the concept of finger sticking and it can really help an individual keep track of sugar patterns.

The most important finger stick of the day is a fasting finger-stick which is taken 8-12 hours after not eating. This number provides a decent estimation of what your body's actual sugar levels are at baseline.

Portion Control

Portion control is an important part of any diet and weight management plan. Our stomachs have adapted to our diet and lifestyle over many years. When you eat a really large meal the diaphragm cannot move as far down, so the lungs do not fill as well. Instead of eating three big meals a day, try dividing your daily food into five or six smaller portions. This way, your stomach will not fill as much after each meal. You can eat a smaller breakfast, lunch and dinner and supply the rest of your nutritional needs for the day by having two or three small snacks.

"

**Sugar?
Nah,
I'm Sweet
enough.**

"

6 | Non-Insulin and Oral Medications

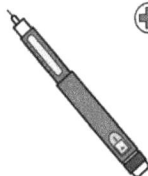

> **"Life** *is a moving, breathing thing.* *We have to be willing to constantly evolve. Perfection is constant transformation."*
>
> *Nia Peeples*

Over the past century advancements of oral diabetic therapy has revolutionized the way we treat diabetes. All oral medications pertain to Type 2 diabetes. The drugs for treating Type 2 diabetes fall into different categories; drugs that increase the amount of natural insulin secreted by beta cells of the pancreas, drugs that increase the sensitivity of target organs to insulin, and medications that decrease the rate at which glucose is absorbed from the gastrointestinal tract. This chapter will outline the different types oral medications available for treatment of Type 2 diabetes.

Biguanides

The main drug in this class is Metformin. It is often considered the first-line drug of choice for the treatment of Type 2 diabetes, in particular, in overweight and obese people as well as those with a normal kidney. The mechanism of action of Metformin is that it suppresses the production of glucose by the liver. In addition Metformin is the only diabetic drug that has shown to prevent the cardiovascular complications of diabetes. Metformin is relatively safe with few known side effects with a low risk of hypoglycemia. If you experience upset stomach or any other side effects please notify your doctor.

Sulfonylureas

Sulfonylureas are a class of diabetic medication that acts by increasing insulin release from the beta cells in the pancreas. They are often the first or second choice of medication in treatment of type 2 diabetes. Examples include: glipizide, glyburide, glimepiride. Since these medications increase insulin production they may induce hypoglycemia. This may occur if the dose is too high or if a patient is fasting and still takes the medication.

Thiazolidinediones

Thiazolidinediones also known as glitazones, are a class of medications also used in the treatment of diabetes mellitus Type 2. These drugs are considered to be insulin sensitizers exerting their effect through the activation of a receptor that decreases insulin resistance. These drugs will make your own natural insulin work more effectively. Some examples of these drugs are as follows. Rosiglitazone (Avndia®) and Pioglitazone (Actos ®). Side effects may include water retention which may aggravate existing heart conditions. If you experience any shortness of breath or chest pain please consult your physician.

Meglitinides

Meglitinides are a class of medications that increase production of insulin from the beta cells in the pancreas. These drugs are rapid acting with half-life of less than 1 hour causing a rapid pulse of insulin making these drugs ideal to take with meals to prevent post prandial hyperglycemia. Examples of these drugs include Repaglinide (Prandin®) and Nateglinide (Starlix®). Side effects include hypoglycemia.

Alpha-glucosidase inhibitors

Alpha-glucosidase inhibitors work by preventing the digestion of carbohydrates and sugars from the digestive tract. These drugs prevent the absorption of the simple sugars from the gut, therefore reducing the blood sugar levels. Examples of these drugs include Acarbose (Precose®), Miglitol (Glyset®) and Voglibose (Voglib®). Side effects include gastrointestinal side effects such as flatulence and diarrhea.

Injectable Incretin Mimetics

Glucagon-like peptide (GLP) agonists – These drugs bind to a receptor increasing insulin release from the pancreatic beta cells. They are normally administered by subcutaneous injection to prevent denaturalization in the digestive tract. Some examples include Exenatide (Byetta®) and Liraglutide (Victoza®).

Dipeptidyl Peptidase-4 Inhibitors

Dipeptidyl peptidase-4 inhibitors work by reducing glucagon which in turn reduces blood sugars Sitagliptin (Januvia®), Saxagliptin (Onglyza®), Linagliptin (Tradjenta ®) and Alogliptin (Nesina®). Some side effects of these medications may include: nasopharyngitis, headache, nausea, hypersensitivity, and skin reactions.

List of Oral Diabetes Medications

Type of Medicine	Route	How They Work	Dosing Schedule
Meglitinides	Oral	Help beta cells release insulin	1-4 times daily
Sulfonylureas	Oral	Help beta cells release insulin	1 or 2 times daily
Biguanides	Oral	Lower sugar production by the liver	1 or 2 times daily
Thiazolidinediones	Oral	Help Cells and tissues use insulin	1 or 2 times daily
Alpha-Glucosidase Inhibitors	Oral	Slow digestion of sugar	Before each meal
GLP-1 agonists	Injectable	Help beta cells release insulin, stop release of un-needed sugar by liver, slow emptying of the stomach	Inject once or twice daily
DPP-4 Inhibitors	Oral	Help beta cells release insulin and decrease glucagon secretion	Once daily

"

FIVE RIGHTS
Right Medication
Right Patient
Right Dose
Right Route
Right Time

"

7 | Insulin Therapy

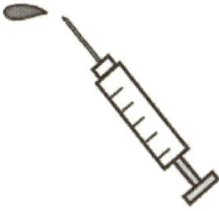

"A mortal lives not through that breath that flows in and that flows out. The source of his life is another and this causes the breath to flow."

Paracelsus (1493-1541)

Insulin is a hormone that is produced by the beta cells in the pancreas. These cells make and release insulin. Beta cells help deliver insulin in the right amount at the right time, such as, when your blood sugar is too high, after meals. As we have learned, insulin therapy is important in all types of diabetes. For Type 1 diabetics it is something they use all the time. For Type 2 diabetics insulin is used when oral medications alone are not controlling the sugar. To properly use insulin it must be injected, because the stomach acids in the digestive system denature the insulin protein.

Type 1 Diabetes

In Type 1 diabetes insulin therapy is the only therapeutic option. Most patients with Type 1 diabetes use at least two types of insulin. The rationale behind this is that there needs to be insulin that creates an increased basal level of insulin in the body, and one type of insulin that is used with each meal to prevent spikes in blood sugars.

Type 2 Diabetes

In the early stages of Type 2 diabetes, diet and exercise may control the sugar alone. However since Type 2 is a progressive disease, medication will have to be added at some point. It is possible that after many years with Type 2 diabetes the pancreas will not be able to supply the body with enough insulin. If this occurs, exogenous insulin will be needed to supplement oral medications. Progression to requiring insulin occurs in about 40% of people with Type 2 diabetes and usually can occur within ten years post diagnosis. With the addition of insulin the dosages of oral medication may have to be changed.

There are different types of insulin. The type varies according to how long before they start and continue to work in your body.

They each have a different:

- Onset of action (when they start to working)
- Time of peak action (when their effect on blood sugar is strongest)
- Duration of action (how long they work)

Fast Acting Insulin

Insulin Aspart (Novolog ®) – this is a rapid acting insulin analogue. It was created using recombinant DNA technology. This type of insulin also prevents the formation of insulin complexes, to create faster acting insulin. Aspart insulin has been approved for use in insulin pumps as well as subcutaneous injection.

Insulin Lispro (Humalog®) – it is a fast acting insulin analogue. This insulin is also made through recombinant DNA technology. The advantage of Insulin Lispro is that it is better for post-prandial glucose control. Its shortened delay of onset allows a little bit more flexibility than that of regular insulin. Both preparations should be coupled with longer acting insulin for good glycemic control.

Insulin glulisine (Apidra®) – it is a fast-acting insulin analogue that differs from human insulin. Due to its quick onset time of approximately 15 minutes, it works after human insulin.

Short Acting Insulin

Regular insulin – Produced by many companies to mimic the body's naturally produced insulin. It is considered to be short acting with an onset time of approximately 30 minutes.

Intermediate Acting Insulin

NPH insulin (Novolin ®, Humalin ®) - is an intermediate-acting insulin given to help control the blood sugar level of those with diabetes. It is a mixture of crystalline zinc insulin combined with a positively charged protein. When it is injected subcutaneously, it has an intermediate duration of action which allows for better glycemic control throughout the day.

Long Acting Insulin

Insulin glargine (Lantus ®) – it is a long-acting basal insulin analogue that is used to control blood sugar levels throughout the whole day. Its mechanism of action mimics the basal insulin secretion of the body's natural pancreatic beta cells. It is used in both Type 1 and Type 2 diabetes. Due to its long acting nature in many patients it must be used in combination with short acting insulin to help meal driven hyperglycemia.

Insulin detemir (Levemir®) – it is a long-acting human insulin analogue for maintaining the body's basal level of insulin. It was has been found that insulin detemir reduced HemoglobinA1c to target levels for majority of patients without as many episodes of hypoglycemia and weight gain.

Combination Insulin

Combination insulin includes a combination of both a shorter acting insulin and longer acting insulin. The combination products begin to work with the shorter acting insulin depending on the specific insulin, and will remain active for 16 to 24 hours. There are several variations with different proportions of the mixed insulin.

How to Take Insulin

Insulin Pen Method

Insulin pens come in two basic styles: disposable and reusable. Disposable pens are pre-filled with insulin, stored in the refrigerator until opened and once opened, are stored at room temperature. When the insulin is used up, the pens are thrown away. Reusable pens are loaded with separately purchased insulin cartridges. The cartridges of insulin are stored in the refrigerator until placed in the pen, but the reusable pen is not refrigerated.

With both types of pens, you screw on a special needle that is thrown away after each use. You dial in a dose, insert the needle into your skin, and press a button to inject the insulin.

Vial and Syringe Method

There are some basic steps involved in giving yourself insulin using the traditional vial and syringe

1. Wash your hands – it is important to prevent any bacteria from entering the breaks in the skin where insulin is injected.
2. Wipe the top of the insulin bottle with an alcohol swab as well as where you plan to inject the insulin to create a sterile environment.
3. Pull back the syringe until it shows the number of units you need.
4. Insert the syringe needle into the top of the insulin bottle and push the plunger forward.
5. Pull back on the syringe plunger until it draws the amount of insulin you need into the syringe.
6. Remove the filled syringe from the bottle. Holding the syringe at a 90-degree angle, insert the needle all the way into your skin and push the plunger forward. If you're thin, it's sometimes easier to inject the insulin at a 45-degree angle.
7. Remove the syringe and dispose safely in a sharps container.

Hypoglycemia

Insulin is very helpful in the setting of diabetes, but it requires close monitoring. If a meal is missed or an accidental overdose of insulin takes place hypoglycemia may occur. Hypoglycemia means low blood sugar. It may occur when you're initially starting to use insulin. There are many signs and symptoms associated with hypoglycemia which are as follows:

- Confusion
- Abnormal behavior
- Double or blurred vision
- Heart palpitations

- Tremor
- Anxiety
- Sweating
- Hunger

If an episode of hypoglycemia occurs, it is important to notify your physician. Your doctor may able to make adjustments to you medications to prevent further episodes of hypoglycemia.

Appendix 4a: List of Insulin Regimen for Diabetes

Insulin Type	When it's usually taken	How soon it starts working	Peak Effect	Duration
Analog Insulin				
Fast Acting	Right before meal	15 min.	30-90 min.	3-5 hr.
Long Acting	30 min. before evening meal or breakfast	1 hr.	Steady over time	Up to 24 hours
Premixed (mix of fast and intermediate acting)	Before breakfast and/or evening meal	5-15 min.	Varies	Up to 24 hours
Human Insulin				
Short Acting	30 min. before meal	30-60 min.	2-4 hr.	5-8 hours
Intermediate Acting (NPH)	30 min before breakfast and/or evening meal	1-3 hr.	8 hours	Up to 24 hours
Premixed (mixture of short (regular) and NPH insulin	30 min before breakfast and/or evening meal	30-60 min.	Varies	Up to 24 hours

"

Soldier in the
INSULIN ARMY
Fighting to
win the war
against
DIABETES

"

8 | Exercise Strategy

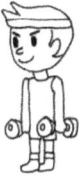

"Walking is man's best medicine."

Hippocrates (460 BC – 377 BC)

Exercise and diabetes go hand in hand socially in terms of managing your diabetes. Exercise can help you improve your blood sugar control and reduce glycated hemoglobin levels. Exercise will also boost your overall fitness and reduce your risk of heart disease and nerve damage.

Measuring Exercise Intensity

It is hard to measure how much energy you are using during the day. In an effort to quantify the energy expenditure of activities of daily living and physical exercise there are some techniques that you can utilize.

- **Talk Test:** The talk test allows you to gauge the intensity of you physical activity. At light intensity a person should be able to sing without any shortness of breath. Moderate exercise a person will be able to carry out a normal conversation. At vigorous intensity a person is too winded to carry out a normal conversation.

- **Heart rate:** This is another way to measure exercise intensity. If your goal is to improve the fitness of your heart and lungs, you should bring your heart rate to a range called the "target heart rate zone." When you stop exercising, quickly take your pulse to find out your heart beats per minute, bpm (see picture). Figure your maximum heart rate by subtracting your age from 220. Your target heart rate zone should be 50 to 75% of your maximum heart rate. So, if you're 50 years old, your maximum heart rate is 170 and your target heart rate zone is 85 to 127.

  My target heart rate range: ....beats per minute (bpm)

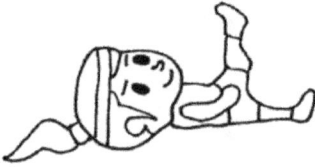

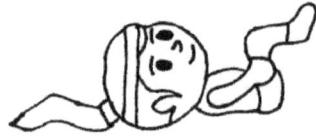

- **Perceived exertion scale:** This is a measurement that allows an individual to assign a numerical value to what a person is feeling in terms of physical stress and fatigue. The scale goes from 6 (at rest) to 20 (maximal exertion)

Exertion Score	Level of Exertion
6	No exertion at all
7-8	Extremely Light
9-10	Very Light
11-12	Light
13-14	Somewhat Hard
15-18	Hard (Heavy)
19	Extremely Hard
20	Maximal Exertion

- **Metabolic Equivalent of Task (MET):** or simply metabolic equivalent was created. This is a measurement expressing the energy cost of physical activities. Below is a table that represents the energy expenditure of daily activities.

Table 3: Representative Levels of Energy Expenditure (in METs)

1.5 – 2 METs	4 – 5 METs
<ul><li>Walking @ 1 mph</li><li>Standing</li><li>Driving automobile</li><li>Sitting at desk or typing</li></ul>	<ul><li>Calisthenics</li><li>Cycling outdoors @ 6 mph</li><li>Golfing (carrying clubs)</li><li>Playing tennis (doubles)</li></ul>
2 – 3 METs	**5 – 6 METs**
<ul><li>Walking at 2.5 – 3 mph</li><li>Dusting furniture, light house work</li></ul>	<ul><li>Walking @ 4 mph</li><li>Digging in garden</li></ul>

	• Ice or roller skating @ 9 mph • Doing carpentry
• Preparing a meal	
3 – 4 METs	6 – 7 METs
• Sweeping • Ironing • Walking 3 mph • Golfing (power cart) • Pushing light lawnmower	• Stationary cycling (vigorous) • Playing Tennis (singles) • Shoveling Snow • Mowing Lawn (non-powered)

Coping with Hypoglycemic Episodes

Once you have spoken to your doctor about exercise and you begin on a exercise regimen, you may find that following the basic advice listed below can help prevent and manage episodes of hypoglycemia.

- It is important that you maintain a structured diet with the same number of meals every day. This will help prevent any spikes or dips in blood sugar.
- Before beginning any form of exercise it is important that you have something to eat to act as fuel for your body. Not eating some carbohydrates before exercising may cause low blood sugar.
- While exercising it is important to stay well hydrated. In addition to water, having a sport drink handy is recommended to replace any electrolytes or water you may have lost during exercise.
- Keeping a supply of glucose tablets at all time is also recommended. Sometimes a sports drink may not be enough to rectify low blood sugars.

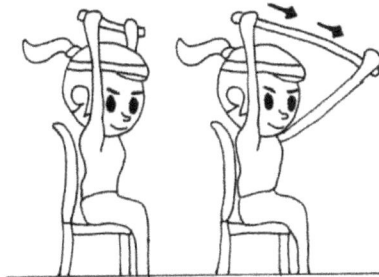

"

The only bad Workout is the One that didn't Happen.

"

9 | Mindfulness

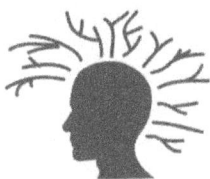

"To keep the body in good health is a duty... otherwise we shall not be able to keep our mind strong and clear."

Buddha (563 BC – 483 BC)

Mind, body and soul are all thought to be connected. It is perceivable that positively affecting anyone of these elements can work for the greater good of your body. In this chapter we will try to pass along tips and guidance to better you mental approach to diabetes management.

Mind Body Activities

Such activities provide a good workout, release tension, and decrease anxiety while promoting health benefits. Yoga, a 5,000 year-old Indian practice, is one such activity and is the best-known mind-body exercise. It involves a series of sitting and laying down postures that help along with coordinated breathing and meditation techniques. Another such technique is Tai Chi, a Chinese method of slow body movement that promotes relaxation. Pilates, like yoga, concentrates on breathing while strengthening the body's core muscles. Meditation can help reduce stress, anxiety and improve quality of life. It is recommended that you get involved in such activities as part of your therapy.

Stress Reduction Techniques - Relaxation and Psychophysical Techniques

The close association between dyspnea and anxiety is well known. If dyspnea is escalated and reinforced by anxiety, as many of you have experienced, a strategy must be developed to reduce the intensity and distress of dyspnea. There are a variety of different techniques that will help you relax during occasions of severe dyspnea and/or anxiety, as well as to decrease stress in daily life. Progressive muscle relaxation is a widely used technique. Some common components of relaxation techniques include the following:

- A quiet environnent
- A confortable position
- Loose and non-restrictive clothes
- Adoption of a passive attitude

Progressive Muscle Relaxation

- Close your eyes.
- Perform 2 large cleansing breaths followed by your pursed-lip breathing.
- With your eyes closed, try to visualize your favorite place to visit. Visualize in your mind the environment, the scenery, the smells and the colors. Try to get in touch with how you feel when you are there. Calm, relaxed and peaceful. Your breathing will begin to slow; you will take slower and deeper breaths.
- Perform slow abdominal breathing with a deep inhalation and a slow exhalation through pursed lips.
- Optional: follow the aforementioned steps followed by systematic tensing then relaxing every part of the body including feet, arms, legs, chest, face, eyes, shoulders, etc., concentrating on each muscle as the tension and relaxation is performed.

Positive Emotion Through Life Skills Training

Appreciate what you already have.

- Once a week write down 5 things that you are thankful for.
- Give thanks for your food and be mindful when you eat.
- Appreciate the beauty in nature.
- Call up people to say thank you for their friendship or care.
- Remember that nothing is guaranteed and nothing lasts forever.
- Look for the good in people.
- Learn to relax, slow down and do one thing at a time, slow and deep diaphragmatic breathing.
- Use a mantra.

Respond appropriately to disappointment.

- Understand that everyone will be disappointed at times. Be prepared by realizing some things will never change. Learn what these are and find the best way for you to work around them.
- All frustrations spring from not getting what you want. Ask yourself if you can control the situation. Don't worry about things that you cannot change.
- Practice forgiveness. Ask yourself, "What am I already doing to solve the problem that does not work.
- You are not alone. Remember that there are many people who have struggled with the same problems you have.

Yoga Exercise

Derived from the Sankrit word "yuj" which means "to unite or integrate"; yoga is a 5,000+ year-old Indian body of knowledge. Yoga is all about harmonizing the body with the mind and breath through the means of various breathing exercises; yoga poses (asanas) and meditation.

Yoga poses are great to strengthen and relax the body, but there is a lot more to it. It is well known that practicing yoga modulates the sympathetic system which controls the release of stress hormone cortisol. Yoga also promotes the parasympathetic branch of the autonomic system which slows down the heart rate and digestion therefore promoting a feeling of calmness and wellness.

There are several types of yoga, but the physical benefits are similar, regardless of the type practiced. Experts say each type of yoga has a slightly different focus, and one may be more appropriate than another for people who have certain interests and abilities.

*Try these set of 12 exercises also referred to as *Surya Namaskar.*

What is Pranayama?

Pranayama are breathing exercises which clear the physical and emotional obstacles in our body to free the breath and the flow of prana - life energy. Through a regular and sustained practice of pranayama you can supercharge your whole body!

By design, nasal breathing and mouth breathing facilitate totally different physiological responses in the body. Breathing through the nose activates the parasympathetic nervous system and mouth breathing encourages the sympathetic nervous system. Your lungs deliver oxygen to your blood. If your lungs can't get enough oxygen to your blood, you can feel short of breath and mouth breathing begins. This elevates the heart rate and encourages the release of more sympathetic hormones into our system.

When we work on the freeing the breath through pranayama (breathing exercises) we are also working on letting the life energy flow through the body. It has the effect of energizing, relaxing, and healing the body; letting everything fall into place.

Pranayama techniques have different effects much like different yoga poses do. Most kinds of pranayama are practiced sitting down with an upright spine, for example in Cross-legged Pose. The idea is for the breath to be smooth and even and not strained even after breath retention.

Some such as Kapalabhati Pranayama (Skull Shining Breath) are energizing and detoxing with a fast rhythm and strong abdominal contractions to expel the breath.

Others are balancing or relaxing like Nadi Shodhana (Alternate Nostril Breathing) or Sama Vritti (Equal Breathing) where inhalations and exhalations are equal length.

10 | Staying Healthy

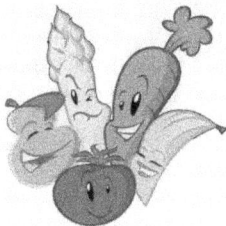

> *"No disease that can be treated by diet should be treated with any other means."*
>
> *Maimonides (1135-1204)*

While your doctor is providing you the best way to manage your disease medically, ultimately you are in charge of your own health. In this section, you'll find practical advice on how to handle your health and other suggestions to make life easier, healthier and more positive.

See your doctor regularly

Even if you're feeling fine, stick to your appointment schedule. Schedule your next appointment while you're at the office, so you won't forget. When you visit your physician in addition to your prescribed medications, please be sure to inform them of any vitamins, herbal supplements, or alternative medicines you may be taking. It is also important to notify your physician of any allergies to food or medications. Common food allergies may include: peanuts, milk, soy, nuts from trees, eggs, and wheat.

Take your medications as prescribed

Bring an updated list of your medication to be reconciled with your chart on every visit. Provide your physicians with a mail order pharmacy number as well as a local pharmacy. If you are using any devices such as a continuous glucose monitoring system (CGMS) or insulin pump, please provide your physician with a number to your medical equipment company. Before you leave your doctor's office make sure your refills have been ordered. You may have more than one medical condition that must be considered when making a dietary plan, so always talk with a healthcare provider or registered dietician before making changes in your diet. Set up a system that will help you remember to take your medications at the appropriate times. On the day of an appointment, schedule time in to take your medications.

Track your condition and symptoms

Prior to coming to your doctor visit you should also write down any questions or topics you want to discuss with your doctor. In diabetes it is imperative that you keep monitoring your blood sugars. It is important to keep a finger stick and food diary. In addition please keep a log of your blood pressure and other vital signs. Make it a point to discuss all of your current and previous lab work. Record dates of all previous diagnostic testing such as echocardiography, stress test and radiological testing.

Quit Smoking

One of the best ways you can make a positive change to your overall health is to quit smoking.

Be active and get stronger

Talk to your doctor about what activities are appropriate to do. With regular exercise, you may find an improvement in your blood sugars, appetite; sleep patterns and your overall sense of well-being. Regular physical activity reduces your risk of heart disease and stroke. It also helps you reduce or control other risk factors such as high blood pressure, high blood cholesterol, excess body weight and diabetes. But the benefits don't stop there. You may look and feel better, become stronger and more flexible, have more energy and reduce stress and tension. The time to start is now.

Exercise regularly

Walking is an excellent activity. Start walking at a slow, comfortable pace for a short period of time (try 5 to 10 minutes) three to five days each week. When you're able to walk the entire time without stopping to rest, you can increase your walking duration by 1 to 2 minutes each week. A sign of a healthy lifestyle is taking 10,000 steps a day. You can monitor your steps per a day by acquiring a pedometer which is available at most sporting or health store. Choose activities you enjoy. Pick a starting date that fits your schedule and gives you enough time to begin your program, like a Saturday. Some tips to help you exercise are:

- Wear comfortable clothes and shoes.
- Start slowly - don't overdo it.
- Try to exercise at the same time so it becomes a regular part of your lifestyle. For example, you might walk every day (during your lunch hour) from 12:00 to 12:30 or start each morning with stretching and strength training.

- Drink lots of water before, during and after each exercise session.
- Ask a friend to start a program with you.
- Note the days you exercise and write down the distance or length of time of your workout and how you feel after each session. You may also want to note if your muscles are tired the next day.
- If you miss a day, plan a make-up day. Don't double your exercise time during your next session.

Have a positive attitude - Try not to compare yourself with others. Your goal should be your own personal health and fitness. Think about whether you like to exercise alone or with other people, outside or inside, what time of day is best and what kind of exercise you most enjoy doing.

- Join a support group
- Join an exercise class
- Exercise with friends or family to help motivate you

Relax - When you feel stressed, consider a stress reduction strategy as discussed later in the chapter.

Maintain a healthy weight - Increased body weight will greater the demand on your heart and lungs. To maintain a healthy weight eat smaller portions, exercise more frequently and discuss with your doctor of medical weight loss management.

Breathe better air - It is important to stay away from cigarette smoking as well as second hand smoke, irritants, mold or any other respiratory triggers. Use an air conditioner and change the air filters frequently to keep the air less humid, cleaner and more comfortable to breathe.

Vaccinations

Vaccines play an important role in health maintenance of patients with advanced lung disease. (See Table)

Flu Vaccine - A seasonal vaccine is distributed routinely every year. Generally everyone 6 months or older should get vaccinated against the flu. Most people who get flu do not need any therapy and generally recover within two weeks. Some people are more likely to get complications like pneumonia, bronchitis, sinus infection and ear infections. The flu can also make chronic health problems like asthma, heart failure, and diabetes worse. Listed below is the group of people more likely to get flu related complications if they get sick from influenza.

Persons at increased risk for flu-related complications include:

- Persons >65 years of age
- Residents of chronic care facilities housing persons of any age with chronic medical conditions
- Persons with chronic cardiopulmonary disease, including children with asthma, COPD
- Persons requiring regular medical care for chronic diseases, including diabetes mellitus, kidney or liver dysfunction, or blood disorders (Sickle cell disease)
- Persons with weakened immune system (e.g. HIV)
- People who are morbidly obese (Body Mass Index >40)
- Health care workers (physicians, nurses) and other people who live or care for high risk people to keep from spreading flu to high risk people

Pneumococcal Vaccine

Pneumonia caused by bacteria *Streptococcus pneumoniae* (pneumococcus) is particularly notorious for causing significant morbidity and mortality. Pneumococcal vaccine is effective at preventing severe disease, hospitalization and death. However, it is not guaranteed to prevent symptomatic infection in everyone. Adults, 65 years of age or older and children younger than 5 years of age are more prone to pneumonia infection. People up to 64 years of age who have underlying medical conditions such as diabetes, HIV/AIDS and people 19 through 64 who smoke or have asthma are also at increased risk for getting pneumonia.

Pneumovax® is 23-valent polysaccharide vaccine (PPVSV) that is currently recommended for use in all adults who are older than 65 years of age and for persons who are 2 years and older and at high risk for disease (e.g., sickle cell disease, HIV infection, or other immuno-compromising conditions like cardiovascular diseases, chronic pulmonary diseases, diabetes mellitus, alcoholism, cirrhosis). It is also recommended for use in adults 19 through 64 years old who smoke or who have asthma.

Varicella Zoster Virus Vaccine

Herpes zoster, commonly known as shingles, is a viral disease characterized by a painful skin rash with blisters in a limited area on one side of the body often in a linear fashion. The initial infection with varicella zoster virus (VZV) causes the acute, short-lived illness chickenpox which generally occurs in children and young adults. The VZV vaccine is recommended by the Centers for Disease Control for any individual over the age of 60.

Tetanus Toxoid Vaccine

Tetanus is a medical condition characterized by prolonged contraction of skeletal muscle. The primary symptoms are caused by tetanospasmin, a neurotoxin produced by the bacteria *Clostridium tetani*. Tetanus infection generally occurs through contamination through an open wound that involves a cut or deep puncture wound. As the infection progresses, muscle spasms develop in the jaw and elsewhere in the body. Most individuals have been vaccinated at one point in their lives but it is recommended that you receive a tetanus booster every 10 years.

Recommended Adult Vaccinations (http://www.cdc.gov)

Vaccine	Age 18-60	Age 60+
Influenza	One dose annually	One dose annually
Varicella	2 doses	
Zoster		1 dose
Pneumococcal poly saccharine (PPSV23)	1 or 2 doses	1 dose (65+)
Pneumococcal 13-valent conjugate (PCV13)	1 dose	
Measles, Mumps, rubella (MMR)	1 or 2 doses	
Meningococcal	1 or more doses	
Hepatitis A	2 doses	
Hepatitis B	3 doses	

Stick to the plan - If you want to optimize your health, stick to your pulmonary treatment, even if it doesn't feel like it's making much of a difference right now stock to your management plan over the course of your treatment, there will be ups and downs. Don't let either success or failure of a treatment to work shake your routine. Follow your treatment plan and if you have a question, discuss it with your doctor.

Stay motivated for optimum health.

- Use a variety of exercises to keep your interest up. For example walk one day, take a swim the next and then go for a bike ride on the weekend.
- Try finding some exercise videos online. Find exercises or style of workouts you find the most interesting.
- Make exercise part of your regular routine so it becomes a habit which you become accustomed to.
- If you take a break from exercising for any length of time, don't lose hope! Just get started again, slowly and work up to your old pace.
- Don't push yourself too hard. You should be able to talk during exercise. Also, if you don't feel recovered within 10 minutes of stopping exercise, you're working too hard.
- If you have heart disease or have had a stroke, members of your family also may be at higher risk. It's very important for them to make changes now to lower their risk.

Blood sugar levels rise and fall throughout the day. By checking your blood sugar you can learn how well your diabetes care plan is working. Understanding why your blood glucose changes can help you to keep your blood glucose on target.

- Eat a well balanced diet as outlined by your nutritionist. A healthy diet for a person with diabetes is a healthy diet for everyone. Avoid foods that are high in fats and simple carbohydrates. Foods to avoid include fruit juices, bagels, pizza and fast food.
- If you have no contraindications (ulcer, bleeding tendency, other blood thinners, etc) take a regular or coated aspirin every day.
- You should have your A1C tested every three months. This test tells how well you've controlled your blood sugar during the past 3 months. An A1C of less than 6.8% is recommended.
- Make sure you know your cholesterol level and have it checked every year. Your LDL or bad cholesterol should be below 100 mg/dl. Your HDL or good cholesterol should be above 40 mg/dl. Your triglycerides should be below 150 mg/dl.
- Keep your blood pressure below 130/80. This will help to keep your heart, kidneys and eyes healthy.

- People with diabetes must see an ophthalmologist for a yearly eye exam. Make sure you tell your eye doctor that you have diabetes.
- You should have a urine test for "microalbumin" (tiny amounts of protein) at least once a year.
- Try to include exercise in your daily routine. You should be exercising at least 30 minutes each day unless otherwise advised.
- Smoking is extremely dangerous for people with diabetes. There are many tools available to help you quit.
- It is important to cook your food fresh and to avoid frozen foods.
- Do not overcook your food as the burning process may create acrylamide which is a known carcinogen.

How can visits with your primary care doctor be helpful?

Visit with your primary care physician are an important part of staying healthy. Many health problems that develop later on in life may be preventive by taking care of your health and keep regular checkups. Physical examination by your primary care physician and routine blood work promotes early detection of the most common yet treatable diseases, such as cancer, diabetes and heart disease.

- Well Visits for Healthy Young Adults (Ages 19-39) should be every 5 years.
- Well Visits for Healthy Adults (Ages 40-49) should be every 1 to 3 years.
- Well Visits for Adults (Ages 50 and Up) should be every 1 to 2 years.

Blood tests that your primary care physician may order

Complete Blood Count (CBC)

The CBC is a test that is ordered to get a profile of the blood cells in your body. The CBC provides information about the white blood cells (WBC), the red blood cell (RBC) and platelets that are in the blood. This information includes the number, type, size, shape and some of the observations of the cells.

- White blood cells (WBC's) protect the body against infection

- Red blood cells (RBC's) carry oxygen
- Platelets help stop bleeding

Lipid Panel (Cholesterol Test)

The Cholesterol test or sometimes called the lipid test, is used to estimate your risk of developing heart disease. Cholesterol is important for your body to produce hormones and help with digestion (The breakdown of food you eat). The fats you eat are stored in the liver and travel through the body along with Cholesterol. Cholesterol particles are made up of proteins and fats that are bound together to form three main types of cholesterol. The Cholesterol test provides information on Low Density Lipoproteins (LDL), High Density Lipoproteins (HDL), Very Low Density Lipoproteins (VLDL) and Triglycerides. LDL is sticky and will stick to your arteries (Arteries are tubes that carries blood through your body, like pipes carry water to parts of your home). Target cholesterol goals are as follows: An LDL of <100 mg/dL, HDL of >40 mg/dL - and Triglycerides <150 mg/dL

- VLDL carries your triglycerides (Fats) to your fat cells.
- LDL is what remains after the fat has been delivered to its destination.
- HDL carries the remaining LDL back to the liver.
- Triglycerides are fats in your blood used to store energy when needed.

Comprehensive Metabolic Panel (CMP)

The CMP is routinely ordered as part of a blood work-up for a medical exam or your yearly physical. The test is usually conducted after you have been fasting. This test will test the electrolytes in your body as well as the liver and kidney function. The test may not tell your physician exactly what is wrong with you, but may give an idea of what may be causing the abnormal test results.

Liver Tests

- ALP (alkaline phosphatase), Bilirubin
- ALT (alanine amino transferase, also called SGPT)
- AST (aspartate amino transferase, also called SGOT)

ALP, ALT and AST are enzymes found in the liver and other tissues. These enzymes are used to determine if your liver is working properly. Bilirubin is a waste product when your liver eliminates old red blood cells.

Other Regular Health Maintenance Testing

- Blood Pressure monitoring and measurement every few months
- Colonoscopy every 5 years
- Eye exam every 2 years (Every one year for Diabetics)
- For women, a pap smear periodically as recommended by OB/GYN.
- For males, Prostate Specific Antigen (PSA) every year.

Check-List for Follow-up Visits of Patients with Diabetes

- Glycemic control: if stable, two to three times per week; but if unstable, two to three times per day.
- Body weight (every month)
- Blood pressure (every month)
- Hemoglobin AA (every three months)
- Urine Analysis (micro-albumin urea) (every 6-12 months)
- Blood urea, serum creatinine, lipid profile (cholesterol, triglycerides, HDLC) (every six months)
- Visual acuity, fundus examination (every 12 months)
- E.C.G. (every 12 months)
- Chest X-ray (at least once)

Tips for choosing a doctor

Choosing a doctor is an important decision that requires research. Ideally, you want a doctor that you are comfortable with and whose skill and instincts you trust. Why is it important to have a doctor that you can be open with? Because when you are able to work as a team with your doctor, you can maximize your ability to fight your disease and stay healthy. Here are some tips for selecting a doctor that can ensure receiving the care that you need and deserve.

- Listening skills - A doctor should treat your medical concerns with careful consideration and not dismiss them. If you feel that he or she is not listening to your chief concerns, then find a doctor that is open to hearing you. You know you body better than anyone else. If something feels abnormal to you, then you need a doctor to take your opinion into account.

- Doctor time - Are you allowed enough time at your appointments to speak directly with your doctor? If you are spending the majority of your time with another clinician (e.g., nurse or physician assistant) and rarely ever see your doctor, then you may not be receiving the attention that you deserve. Nurses are incredibly knowledgeable, but there should also be an adequate amount of direct "face time" with your doctor.

- Responsiveness - An unresponsive doctor is not someone that is going to be attentive to your needs. If he or she doesn't return calls or faxes, find a clinician that can. Having your questions answered in a timely manner is crucial to identifying a problem at the earliest stage. Response time is critical to protecting your health.

- Familiarity - During follow-up appointments, is your doctor knowledgeable about major events in your medical history? It may not be critical that he or she remember every single past issue, but you doctor should be aware of significant events in your life and medical history. If it feels like that first meeting each time you see your doctor, then you may want to consider someone that can provide you with the utmost in care.

11 | Complications of Diabetes

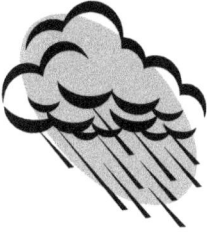

"The biggest disease this day and age is that of people feeling unloved."

Princess Diana (1961-1997)

Diabetes is dubbed the "silent killer" as sugars can remain elevated without any specific symptoms. However, when sugars remain elevated for an extended period of time it may cause complications. All complications of diabetes are associated with elevated sugars. This chapter will outline the complications that are commonly seen in the settings of diabetes.

Diabetes increases the risk of many serious complications. These complications are divided into two categories: Microvascular (affecting small vessels) and Macrovascular (affecting large vessels). Liver and muscles are main storage sites for sugar. Any excess amount of sugar that is not absorbed can move around and damage nerves and blood vessels. It is unfortunate that sugars can affect almost every major organ in the body, i.e. brain, heart, kidney. Once a patient is diagnosed with diabetes, controlling your blood sugars becomes an important objective. Even though you are feeling fine, treatment of DM2 can't be ignored. Many of the effected organs are affected gradually over a period 10-20 years and can eventually lead to disabling or even life threatening conditions.

Diabetes and Heart Disease

Cardiovascular disease (CVD) is the most common long-term complications of uncontrolled diabetes. The risk of CVD is two to four times greater in patients with diabetes than in non-diabetic patients and they develop it at an earlier age. High sugar levels damage lining of blood vessels and making it harder for blood vessels to pump blood throughout the body, as a result, increasing the force to move blood throughout the body. This refers to as hypertension. In addition, high sugars cause an imbalance between good cholesterol (HDL) and bad cholesterol (LDL) as well as high levels of triglycerides. This buildup, referred to as 'plaque' can also cause the heart to pump with higher pressure.

Hypertension or high blood pressure is an important factor in diabetes. It puts a strain on your heart and increases your chance of a heart attack. In many cases, people aren't even be aware that they maybe hypertensive. Patients can sometime present without any symptoms of chest pain. There are some diagnostic tests available to monitor your heart are EKG, Echocardiogram and Cardiac stress. For a diabetic patient, blood pressure should be <130/80 mmHg. Along with weight loss, low salt intake, medications are available to control your blood pressure. ACE inhibitors are usually the first recommended medication. Other medications available include: ARBs, Beta blockers, diuretics and calcium channel blockers. The patient should also control blood lipid concentration with a target of LDL< 100 mg/dl. In patient with CVD, the target LDL should be <70 mg/dl. Any patient with LDL >100 should be considered for drug therapy. If patient has LDL>130, statin therapy is a must.

Diabetes and Kidney Disease (Diabetic Nephropathy)

The kidneys are a remarkable organ. They are made of small tiny units called nephrons that are surrounded by tiny blood vessels called capillaries. These vessels bring in blood filled with nutrients and toxins. The function of kidney is to filter all toxins and harmful substances from our body and reabsorb essential nutrients that were filtered along with it. If blood sugars are uncontrolled, these tiny blood vessels are damaged and leak materials that may be necessary for body. Eventually the kidneys stop working and can cause kidney failure. There are instances in which protein loss can occur but only temporarily, i.e. during exercise, heart failure, or illness.

Certain risk factors place a patient in high risk category to have kidney damage. If a person has history of prior smoking, high blood pressure or high cholesterol, he/she is at risk of having kidney problems in the future. Patients from certain ethnic groups such as Pima Indians in Arizona, African-Americans and Hispanics are more prone to developing kidney problems.

Factors associated with diabetic nephropathy are:

- Glycemia
- Diabetes duration
- Hypertension
- Hyperfiltration
- Ethnicity
- Genetics
- Diet (protein intake)

Diabetic nephropathy requires a clinical diagnosis. Abnormalities in the kidney can first be seen when some amount of protein is lost in the urine. This can be detected by a simple urine test. Damage to the kidney may not appear immediately. The kidneys have a massive network of filtering capability that more than 60% of function must be lost before any damage can be observed. Hence, it takes about 5 to 10 years after being diagnosed with diabetes to observe any change in kidney function. Patients with kidney disease may complain of nausea, headache, leg swelling. Doctors can order certain tests that will assess the function of kidney and manage accordingly.

The first test to detect any damage is called microabluminuria (once a year) to see if any protein was lost in urine. A positive test occurs if the value > 30ug/mg and will require very strict sugar control. Tight glycemic control helps control amount of damage to kidney. Without any aggressive treatment, this protein loss can gradually worsen leading to increase blood pressure and eventually lead to ERSD. If the kidneys stopped working, then the patients rely on a dialysis machine to do the work of kidneys. However, dialysis may be the only option for some patients. Diabetes is the single most common reason for ESRD that will require renal transplant.

Two tests done annually patients should undergo to check status of kidney:

- Urine test for protein (microalbumin)
- Blood test for creatinine (waste product of metabolism)

Once it is confirmed that there is some protein loss, physicians can start medications that will slow down progression of kidney damage. The cornerstone of therapy is starting patients on ACE inhibitors/ARBs to control blood pressure because even a small rise in blood pressure can drastically affect kidney function.

Apart from medication, there are certain things that need to be done to protect your kidneys. Any diagnostic imaging tests, such as MRI, CT scan that require a contrast medium and medications such as NSAIDs should be avoided. A low protein diet along with low sodium diet should be started.

Diabetes and Nerve Disease (Diabetic Neuropathy)

Diabetic neuropathy is a term that includes an assorted group of disorders. The nervous system is essentially made of circuits that controls all our daily actions such walking, eating and breathing, regardless of being awake or asleep. All the input is sent from distant extremities to the brain and it analysis this information and sends a response. Tiny blood vessels are supplying these nerves with nutrients including sugars. Nearly 50% of diabetics are affected by an excess amount of sugar, as a result, hindering the normal function and impeding transfer of information. Evaluation of any neuropathy involves a complete history and physical examination that documents any changes in sensation patients have noticed. If they have noticed, doctors can explore further about duration, location and how long they have had these deficits.

Diabetic neuropathy is divided into sub categories: peripheral (nerves outside of brain and spinal cord), autonomic (involuntary nerves) proximal, or focal. Each affects different parts of the body in various ways.

Peripheral Neuropathy:

Peripheral Neuropathy is also referred to as distal symmetric neuropathy. This type of neuropathy involves damage that begins at feet and later spreads to the hands. Patients may feel some burning, numbness and tingling sensation, as a result of damage, in a symmetrical pattern. This is also referred to as "Stocking/glove pattern." Patient can also feel pain on light touch "burning" pain that can be unbearable to tolerate and are worst at night. The main concern is that people may not realize they have some nerve problems.

The loss of sensation can lead to:

- Ulcer formation because patients don't' shift their weight.
- Stepping on sharp objects without noticing.
- Small blisters/cuts may go unnoticed and worsen over time.
- Patients can't tell difference between hot or cold if they touch anything.
- May affect patient's gait (walking)
- Developing ingrown toe nails leading to infection.

People with diabetes are prone to having some foot problems and therefore taking care of the feet requires extra effort. The damage caused by high sugars can be significant enough to cause ulcers and infections in patient's feet. Patients with diabetes are prone to dry and cracked skin allowing bacteria to grow resulting in serious bacterial infections. Other problems that can occur include: bunions, corns, calluses, and ingrown toenails.

Calluses and corns are thickened areas of skin that occur between toes due to high pressure created by high heels or narrow shoes. In Diabetes patients, these areas present as site of ulcer formation (open wound). Nerve damage causes loss of sensation and patients should not cut the calluses on their own by knives or blades because that can lead to serious infection. Using a pumice stone can help control calluses formation. Visiting a health care provider (podiatrist) is important and they are trained professional to cut any excess calluses. Avoiding tight fitting shoes or having extra foot pads can help reduce calluses.

Other Tips to keep feet infection free:

- Never walk barefoot. Wear shoes and socks of appropriate size. Wear only comfortable shoes with soft socks made of wool or cotton. Avoid wearing tight pointed shoes or flip flops.
- Check feet daily to notice any sores or cuts. Ask for assistance from family member.
- Keep feet clean with warm water and dry them using a soft towel.

- At night, keep feet warm by wearing socks. Don't use heating pads or hot water bottles on feet because they can cause burns.
- Visit your doctor (podiatrist) for regular check on feet.

Diabetes and Eyes Disease (Diabetic Retinopathy)

Diabetes affects blood vessels in the eyes and is a leading cause of blindness in United States. It mainly affects the retina, iris, and lens.

Cataracts refer to clouding of the eye lens that blocks vision. Cataracts are common in old age, but diabetic patients are at a greater risk of cataracts. Patients can have decreased or blurred vision that can significantly impair their activities. Patients undergo surgery to remove the cloudy cataract that is replaced by a clear clean artificial lens.

Glaucoma refers to high pressure inside the eye that builds up because it can't be drained properly. This increase in pressure causes nerve and blood vessel damage affecting vision. Fortunately, several medical treatments are available to relieve pressure.

Diabetes Retinopathy: This refers to changes that take place in the retina. These changes are a result of high sugars that weaken the blood vessel wall. As these walls become weak, they may start leaking fluid or even bleed. In some patients, vessels in the eye may swell like a balloon (called micro aneurysms) and in others new blood vessels may grow because old vessels may be damaged by high sugars. These newly made vessels are weak and can break easily. This can effect vision poorly and lead to blindness.

It is important to note that disease may be progressing while the vision is good, regular check up with an eye doctor is important. Doctors will dilate the eye and examine the back of the eye more efficiently and it's completely painless. In addition, keeping control of sugars, and blood pressure as close to normal as possible is beneficial.

Diabetes and other Complications

Oral Cavity/Mouth Complications

Diabetic patients are at higher risk for oral disease. High sugar can cause dental caries, gingivitis or periodontitis.

Dental caries are a result of sugar that can sticks to the tooth forming plaques. The plaque can build up resulting in cavities and cause erosion of the enamel. The plaque can also accumulate in the gum and causing irritation and bleeding (gingivitis). Plaque buildup can also result in tooth loss, destruction of bone that can require major procedures to restore aesthetics.

To avoid oral problems:

- Keep sugar under control.
- Visit dentist or hygienist twice in a year.
- Brushing and/or flossing after eating or at twice a day (morning and before bedtime).
- Ask for guidance for appropriate technique for brushing and flossing.
- Quit smoking
- Check mouth everyday for any changes such as swelling, bleeding etc. If any changes occur, make an appointment with your dentist.

Diabetic Skin Disease

Acanthosis nigricans: dark, brown velvety areas of the body that are result of access pigment deposited in back of the neck, armpits and/or groin. There is no specific treatment for this, except sugar control.

Diabetes and Foot Care

One very susceptible part of the body in the setting of diabetes and elevated sugar levels are the nerves of the peripheral body, most importantly the feet. Damage to the nerves begins with parathesia (pins and needles sensation) in the feet. Eventually the nerves are destroyed which results in a total loss of sensation. Foot care is very important for all diabetics as lack of care can lead to more severe complications.

It is important to note that diabetes may also affect the small blood vessels in your feet as well as your nerves. When nerve damage occurs it prevents from feeling any pain that may be associated with a cut, scrape or infection. With damage to the blood vessels there is a chance that wounds may not heal as quickly as possible.

Some common conditions seen in diabetics are:

- Bunions
- Corns and calluses
- Blisters
- Dry and cracked skin
- Changes in color of skin
- Athlete's foot
- Hammertoes
- Plantar warts
- Ulcers (open sores)

To ensure that your feet are always as healthy as can be you should follow with a podiatrist (foot doctor) yearly for a checkup. A foot exam will help you to know if you are at risk for foot problems.

Some tips you can follow to keep your feet healthy are:

- Wash your feet every day with warm soap and water
- Do not soak your feet as this will dry out your skin.
- Make sure to dry your feet, even between your toes.
- Put lotion on your feet to prevent dryness or cracking.
- Check your feet every day for open sores, blisters and changes in the shape and color of your skin.
- Be sure to cut your toenails straight across
- Use a nail file to shape and file the edges of the toenails. This will help prevent ingrown nails.

Some advice about proper footwear is:

- Proper fitting shoes can prevent pressure point injury.
- Make sure your shoes are debris free, shake your shoes before you put them on to be sure nothing is inside.
- Wear new shoes for only a few hours and gradually break them in. Interchange with older shoes to prevent any irritation and/or injury.

- Be sure your shoes are comfortable and fit well and have extra depth and width.

Claudication (Peripheral Vascular Disease)

Claudication is the medical term for pain in the leg due to a lack of enough blood flow to the leg. This is due to narrowing of the arteries going to your legs. This may be worsened by diabetes. Symptoms typically include leg pain that worsens with walking and improves with rest. When the pain begins to occur at rest (when no activity or exercise is being performed), it is a sign of severe narrowing of the arteries.

Claudication is a serious condition that is due to narrowing of the blood vessels that supply you leg with blood. It also implies that you may have severe narrowing of other blood vessels in your body, such as in the arteries that supply your heart or your brain. This is sometimes called "hardening of the arteries." This can be tested by performing a Doppler study of the leg arteries. Follow-up with a vascular surgeon is recommended if needed.

If any of the following occurs you should seek medical attention:

- Pain in your legs when at rest.
- Any coolness in the feet or leg.
- Any color changes, especially if one leg looks paler than the other.
- Any other worsening symptoms or concerns.

Impotency and Sexual Health

In addition to all above complications, sexual health in males is affected as well. The microvasculature and neurons that provide the male genitalia are damaged by the increases sugars in the blood. It is important to remember that sex is an important part of social life, marriage and relationships. Diabetes and its complications can disturb this whole aspect of a relationship and can be caused on either or both partners feel there is trouble. Discuss this with one another, as it is important to keep each other informed about your feelings. Remember having diabetes doesn't mean that sexual activity must be reduced, curtailed or totally eliminated.

"

**Please don't
sugar coat it...
I'm a diabetic.**

"

12 | Managing Diabetes at Home

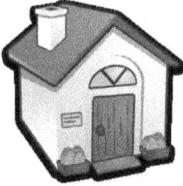

"We are not victims of aging, sickness and death. These are part of scenery, not the seer, who is immune to any form of change. This seer is the spirit, the expression of eternal being."

Deepak Chopra (b. 1947)

To help manage your disease you should first talk to your family members about what you need to do. In addition it is important that you discuss your health issues with your family. Hiding your diagnosis may prevent your family from understanding what you are going through or the support you need. Begin by reviewing the following information. Together, talk to the doctor or nurse about keeping an adequate supply of prescription medications on hand as well as all your diabetic supplies.

Always be prepared:
- You should always have adequate supply of routine medications. In addition, set aside medications to treat episodes of hypoglycemia.
- Identify a health care agent (family member or friend) or a proxy to help make emergent medical decisions.
- Make sure your durable medical devices (insulin pump, continuous glucose monitoring system) are always in working order.
- All important medical and family phone numbers should be on the refrigerator and easy to find.

Tips for Coping with Diabetes

- Make duplicates of all keys. Bury a house key in a secret spot in the garden or carry a duplicate car key in your wallet, apart from your key ring.
- Practice preventive maintenance. Your car, appliances, home and relationships will be less likely to break down/fall apart "at the worst possible moment."
- Procrastination is stressful. Whatever you want to do tomorrow, do today, whatever you want to do today, do it now.
- Allow 15 minutes of extra time to get to appointments.
- Ask questions. Taking a few moments to repeat back directions, what someone expects of you, etc. can save hours.

By keeping track of basic information, you will be able to provide the doctor with accurate and up-to-date reports, either over the phone or during visits. This record does not need to be complicated. In fact, the simpler, the better. A spiral-bound notebook or composition book will do just fine. Have your loved one get in the habit of routinely recording the following information:

- Precipitating factors of shortness of breath (walking, stair climbing, anxiety, upper respiratory infections, etc.)
- List of medications-names, doses, list of all allergies.
- Other symptoms to discuss with your doctor, such as daily weight and leg swelling.
- Swollen hands, ankles, or feet.
- Increased fatigue, chest pain, fainting spells, sleep disruption.
- Shortness of breath that interrupts sleep.

Traveling With Diabetes

As with any other aspect of living with diabetes, planning ahead and taking precaution can allow you to travel with a free mind. It's good to get out of the house and enjoy life. If you can manage diabetes well at home then you should try hard to manage it equally well away from home as well.

What precautions should I take when traveling?

- When you travel alone make sure you travel light and have the appropriate luggage. Always travel with your complete identification including medical information (medical alert bracelet, device identification card, etc)
- Make you sure you keep your cell phone with you at ALL times. This may your only lifeline to call for help if need be.
- Travel at times when traffic is light to cut down travel time.
- On long trips every hour you should exercise your legs to prevent blood clots from forming.
- Stay hydrated by drinking non-alcoholic, non-caffeinated beverages.
- When making hotel reservations or other accommodation, make sure your needs are met (elevators, ramps, etc.)
- Before traveling to a particular city make a list of clinics, hospitals and health centers that will be close to where you are staying.
- If possible, book direct flights. This allows you to avoid any layovers where oxygen may not be available.
- Have your immunizations up to date. Keep a current list of your medications while traveling.
- In addition keep an extra supply of your medications. Bring enough medication to cover your needs in case of a long delay or lost bags.
- Check your health insurance coverage and travel insurance policy to make sure that any medical costs that may arise will be covered.
- Bring the phone numbers of your health care providers, including your physician, respiratory therapist and oxygen supplier.
- Vacations generally involve more walking than you usually do. Check your feet from blisters and sore spot each night.
- Do not forget to check your blood sugars regularly.
- If you use a CPAP machine it is advisable to take a note from your physical about it.

Anyone whose diabetes requires insulin may need additional documentation for the airlines. Medical supplies are available and most countries. Still it is prudent to know the alternative names of generic medications in the country that you are travelling.

Generally airline food is not a problem, unless and until you are on the very strict diet. Please inform the airlines about it while making reservations. A few traveling through several times zones, and he may need to adjust her eating and insulin. Please discuss with your physician before starting your journey. Your physician can help to plan for these adjustments. Sitting on a plane long hours can impede the separation in the veins of the leg. It is important that every few hours you must get up and walk, flex your leg muscles and toes.

Diabetes kills more Americans every year than AIDS and breast cancer combined.

A person with diagnosed diabetes at age 50 dies six years earlier than a counterpart without Diabetes

---

13 | Diabetes & Sleep

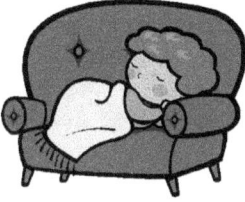

"The good physician treats the disease; the great physician treats the patient who has the disease."

Sir William Osler (1849-1919)

Sleep is an integral part of homeostasis. Without proper sleep, the body's metabolic function is in a sluggish state which may contribute to obesity as well as worsening of diabetes. In this chapter we would like to outline the co-morbidities associated with poor sleep.

Sleep Disorders and Diabetes

The human body needs sleep for recovery and restitution. It is an active state essential for mental and physical restoration. Regular inability to get a good night's sleep may be indicative of a sleep disorder.

Obstructive Sleep Apnea (OSA)

Obstructive Sleep Apnea is the most common sleep disorder. It has been recognized that untreated OSA may lead to an increase in blood sugar levels due to an increase in insulin resistance. It has been established that that adults who suffer from OSA are three times more likely to also have diabetes. It is also known that someone afflicted with both diabetes and sleep apnea is more likely to suffer a stroke in the future. It is also a serious and potentially life-threatening condition that often goes undiagnosed. Loud snoring may signal that something is wrong with breathing during sleep and reflect presence of OSA. The condition affects at least 2-4% of middle-aged adults. Approximately 95% of the affected population remains undiagnosed and untreated.

Some of the warning signs of OSA are, but not limited to excessive daytime fatigue and sleepiness, snoring, falling asleep at inappropriate times, poor performance at home or at work and cessation of breathing at night.

What are the Consequences of Untreated OSA?

When OSA goes untreated it may lead to elevations in blood pressure, heart arrhythmias or even heart failure, poor oxygenation, heart attack, cardiovascular accidents such as stroke, and an increase in insulin resistance. Excessive daytime sleepiness and fatigue may lead to traffic and industrial accidents.

How can Obstructive Sleep Apnea be Treated?

Currently there are a few options for the treatment of OSA. The most effective option is a continuous positive air pressure (CPAP) machine which uses air to help keep your airways open while you sleep. Those who are intolerant to the CPAP device may be considered for surgery or an oro-dental device. The most conservative treatment option is weight loss in conjunction with lifestyle modification. You are encouraged to discuss these therapeutic options with your physician if you suspect you may have OSA symptoms or you have been diagnosed to have OSA. Treatment of OSA with a CPAP machine may improve or help control your diabetes. Research has shown that patients using CPAP therapy for at least four hours a night have significantly lower blood sugars after meals.

How can you measure your daytime sleepiness symptoms?

Johns et al. from Australia devised a screening questionnaire called the Epworth Sleepiness Scale Score to gauge daytime sleepiness. It is a set of questions that assesses your likelihood of falling asleep during daytime situations.

Epworth Sleepiness Scale Score:

0 = Would never doze off
1 = Slight chance of dozing off
2 = Moderate chance of dozing off
3 = High chance of dozing off

_____ Sitting and reading

_____ Watching television
_____ Sitting, inactive in a public place (i.e., movie theater)
_____ Sitting talking to someone
_____ As a passenger in a car for an hour without a break
_____ Sitting quietly after lunch without alcohol
_____ Lying down to rest in the afternoon if time permitted
_____ In a car, while stopped for a few minutes in traffic
_____ **Total Score**

Johns MW. A new method for measuring daytime sleepiness: the Epworth sleepiness scale. Sleep. 1991 Dec; 14(6):540-5.

If your total score is higher than 10, it may indicate excessive daytime sleepiness which is a sign of possible OSA. You should discuss this with your physician to determine whether or not you may have a sleep disorder. Based on this simple questionnaire a health care provider such as a pulmonologist can better gauge if you are a candidate for a sleep study

Another questionnaire to help you gauge the likelihood of you having OSA is the STOP-Bang Questionnaire. This predicts presence of sleep apnea. Answering Yes to 3 or more questions in this questionnaire indicates high probability of presence of OSA.

STOP - Bang Scoring Model

1. Snoring
Do you snore loudly (loud enough to be heard through closed doors)?
.   Yes   No

2. Tired
Do you often feel tired, fatigued or sleepy during daytime?
         Yes   No

3. Observed
Has anyone observed you stopping breathing during your sleep?
         Yes   No

4. Blood pressure
Do you have or are you being treated for high blood pressure?
         Yes   No

5. BMI
BMI more than 35kg/m²?

        Yes   No

6. Age
Age over 50 years old?

        Yes   No

7. Neck circumference
Neck circumference greater than 40?

        Yes   No

8. Gender
Gender male?

        Yes   No

Chung, F., Yegneswaran, B., Liao, P., Chung, S. A., Vairavanathan, S., Islam, S., Khajehdehi, A. and Shapiro, C. M. STOP Questionnaire A Tool to Screen Obstructive Sleep Apnea. Anesthesiology 108, 812-821. 2008.

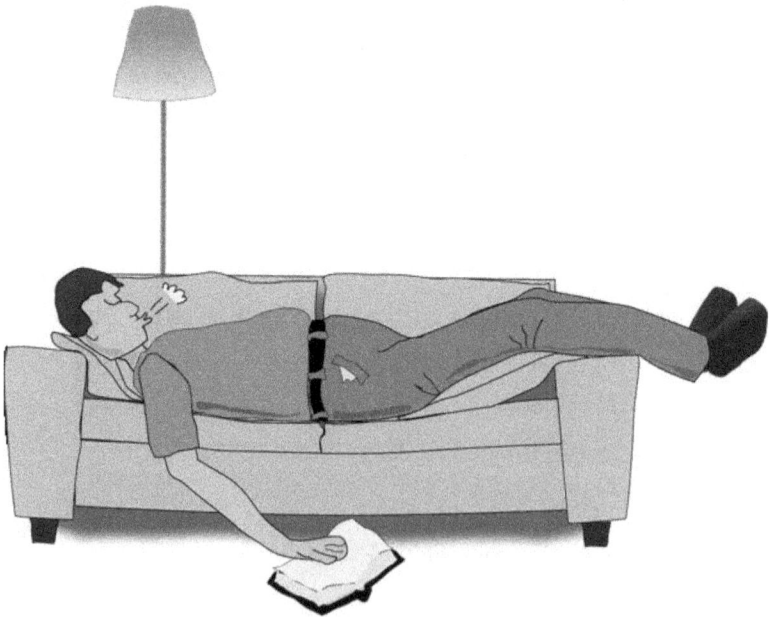

Sleep Hygiene

Poor sleep habits (referred to as hygiene) are among the most common problems encountered in our society. We stay up too late and get up too early. We interrupt our sleep with drugs, chemicals, and work. On top of this we over-stimulate ourselves with late-night activities such as television. Below are some essentials of good sleep habits. Many of these points will seem like common sense. But it is surprising how many of these important points are ignored by many of us.

Your Personal Habits

- Fix a bedtime and an awakening time. Do not be one of those people who allow bedtime and awakening time to drift. The body "gets used" to falling asleep at a certain time, but only if this is relatively fixed. Even if you are retired or not working, this is an essential component of good sleeping habits.
- Avoid napping during the day. If you nap throughout the day, it is no wonder that you will not be able to sleep at night. The late afternoon for most people is "sleepy time". Many people will take a nap at that time. This is generally not a bad thing to do, provided you limit the nap to 30-40 minutes and can sleep well at night.
- Avoid alcohol 4-6 hours before bedtime. Many people believe that alcohol helps them sleep. While alcohol has an immediate sleep-inducing effect, a few hours later as the alcohol levels in your blood start to fall, there is a stimulant or wake-up effect.
- Avoid caffeine 4-6 hours before bedtime. This includes caffeinated beverages such as coffee, tea and many sodas, as well as chocolate, so be careful. Avoid heavy, spicy, or sugary foods 4-6 hours before bedtime. These can affect your ability to stay asleep. Exercise regularly, but not right before going to bed. Regular exercise, particularly in the afternoon, can help deepen sleep. Strenuous exercise within the 2 hours before bedtime, however, can decrease your ability to fall asleep.
- Exercise a digital curfew. Ban digital devices from the bedroom. Technology can alienate people. As smart phones continue to burrow their way into our lives, wearable devices such as Google Glass® threaten to invade out personal space even further.

Your Sleeping Environment

- Use comfortable bedding. Uncomfortable bedding can prevent good sleep. Evaluate whether or not this is a source of your problem and make appropriate changes.
- Find a comfortable temperature setting for sleeping and keep the room well ventilated. If your bedroom is too cold or too hot, it can keep you awake. A cool (not cold) bedroom is often the most conducive to sleep.
- Reserve the bed for sleep. Don't use the bed as an office, workroom or recreation room. Let your body know that the bed is associated with sleeping.

Getting Ready For Bed

- **Eat Light:** Try a light snack before bed. Warm milk and foods high in the amino acid tryptophan, such as bananas, may help you to sleep.
- **Develop a Routine:** Practice relaxation techniques before bed. Relaxation techniques such as yoga, deep breathing and other may help relieve anxiety and reduce muscle tension.
- **Keep a To Do List:** Don't take your worries to bed. Leave your worries about job, school, daily life, etc., behind when you go to bed. Some people find it useful to assign a "worry period" during the evening or late afternoon to deal with these issues.
- **Establish a Pre-sleep Ritual:** Pre-sleep rituals, such as a warm bath or a few minutes of reading, can help you sleep.
- **Find a Sleeping Position:** If you don't fall asleep within 15-30 minutes, get up, go into another room and read until sleepy.
- **Power Down:** Any device with a screen (TV, tablet PC, laptop, iPad) emits a blue spectrum light that can inhibit the brain production of melatonin that induces sleep. Some people find that the radio helps them go to sleep. Since radio is a less engaging medium than TV, this might be a better idea.

Getting Up in the Middle of the Night

Most people wake up one or two times a night for various reasons. If you find that you get up in the middle of night and cannot get back to sleep within 15-20 minutes, then do not remain in the bed "trying hard" to sleep. Get out of bed, leave the bedroom, read, have a light snack, do some quiet activity or take a bath. You will generally find that you can get back to sleep 20 minutes or so later. Do not perform challenging or engaging activity such as office work, housework, etc. Do not watch television.

A Word About Sleeping Aids

Sometimes you may not have any sleep disorder but may find it hard to fall asleep. Make it a point to discuss with your physicians about sleeping aids. Common supplements for sleeping are Valerian root, melatonin and ashwagandha root. Pharmaceutical options for sleeping aids are zolpidem (Ambien®), eszopiclone (Lunesta®), zaleplon (Sonata®) or ramelteon (Rozerem®) also may help you get to sleep. Please discuss all options with your physician.

"

**A good laugh
And a long sleep
Are the two
Best cures for
ANYTHING.**

"

14 | Diabetes and Obesity

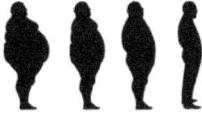

"Weight loss is more than a physical challenge, it's a mental challenge."

LouisKhalido

Obesity

Obesity has recently been recognized by the American Medical Association as a diseased state. Inactivity and a sedentary lifestyle may contribute to obesity and development or worsening of diabetes. Obesity is measure in terms of body mass index (BMI) that is defined as you weight in kilograms divided by you height in meters squared. Below you will find a chart that summarizes the severity of obesity.

Where you carry your body weight also makes a difference. Excess abdominal fat (central or visceral obesity), which is found above the waist, is related to increased risk of diabetes and heart disease. In men a waist greater than 40 inches and in women more than 36 inches is of concern. Fat that accumulates under the skin or in area like the hips and thighs poses less of a health risk.

The following chart illustrates what that number means:

Table 5: Definition of Body Mass Index (BMI)

Body Mass Index (BMI)	Classification	What It Means
Less than 18.5	Underweight	Increased risk of health problems associated with underweight, such as inadequate nutrition.
18.5-24.9	Normal	Healthy body weight for height.

25-29.9	Overweight	Heavier than the optimal for height— carries an increased risk of weight-related health problems.
30-34.9	Obesity I	High risk of common medical problems associated with obesity, such as type 2 diabetes, high blood pressure, abnormal cholesterol and breathing disorders. In most people, a BMI of 30 means they're about 30 to 40 pounds overweight.
35-39.9	Obesity II	Very high risk of common medical problems associated with obesity such as type 2 diabetes, high blood pressure, abnormal cholesterol and breathing disorders.
40 or greater	Obesity III (severe obesity; previously referred to as morbid obesity).	Extremely high risk of associated medical problems. People with a BMI of 40 or greater are typically 100 pounds overweight or more.

Table 6: Risk level associated with waist circumference

	Risk Level	
Category	Healthy	High
Men	≤ 40"	> 40"
Women	≤ 35"	>35"

Management of obesity is centered on weight loss. There are a few options on how to approach this. The first is lifestyle modification that entails changing diet and incorporating exercise into your daily routine. There needs to be a reduction in the net calories that you're consuming to begin weight loss. In cases where lifestyle modification does not help there are pharmaceutical interventions that may kick start your metabolism. These drugs are phentermine/topiramate (Qsymia®), locaserin (Belviq®) and tetrahydrolipstatin (Orlistat®) which work suppressing appetite. For a select few patients where the above two options do not work surgical intervention may be necessary. Please consult with your physician regarding your weight loss options.

Metabolic Syndrome

Metabolic syndrome is a condition defined as a cluster of three or more of the following risk factors in adults:

- Increased abdominal fat: waist circumference in a woman of at least 35 inches, or 40 inches or greater in a man
- Elevated blood pressure on several measurements: 130 or greater systolic (top number) or 85 or greater diastolic (bottom number)
- Elevated level of triglycerides (blood fats): greater than 150 after a twelve-hour fast
- Low level of high-density lipoprotein (HDL)- the "good" cholesterol: under 40 for a man or less than 50 for a woman
- Elevated blood sugar: 110 or greater after a twelve-hour fast—for instance, first thing in the morning, before breakfast; this includes blood sugars in the pre-diabetes range

If you have metabolic syndrome, you face an increased chance of developing cholesterol deposits in the arterial walls (*atherosclerosis*), which causes most heart attacks, strokes, and also provides an increased risk for developing diabetes. Metabolic syndrome occurs in only 5 percent of adults of normal weight, but in 22 percent of those who are overweight and in 60 percent of those who are obese! For these people, the most important interventions are weight loss and exercise.

"

**Lose the inches
lower your risk
tell diabetes,
NOT ME.**

"

15 | Diabetes and Other Health Problems

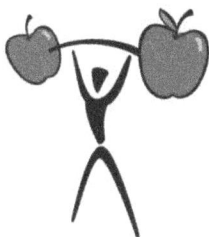

"Our own physical body possesses a wisdom which we who inhabit the body lack. We give it orders which make no sense.

Henry Miller

High blood pressure (Hypertension)

Blood pressure is the force of blood pushing against the inside of your blood vessels, called arteries, as your heart pumps. High blood pressure is a serious condition that causes your heart to work harder. It is also called hypertension. It can cause heart disease, stroke, kidney failure, blood vessel disease and other health problems. Those who are more likely to have high blood pressure include:

- African Americans
- Men over the age of 45 and women over the age of 55
- People with a family history of high blood pressure
- Women who are pregnant, or who take birth control pills, or hormone replacement therapy
- People with health conditions like thyroid disease, chronic kidney disease, or sleep apnea
- Those who take certain medicines, such as asthma medicines and cold-relief products

Your chances of having high blood pressure increase if you:

- Are overweight
- Eat foods high in salt
- Do not get regular exercise
- Smoke
- Drink alcohol heavily

There is no way to tell that you have high blood pressure. The only way to know if you have high blood pressure is to have it checked. The following are some key points regarding your blood pressure measurement:

- There are two blood pressure numbers. Systolic (top number) - the pressure when your heart pumps the blood out of your body.
- Diastolic (bottom number) - the pressure when your heart is resting in between beats.
- Your blood pressure should be less than 120/80 mmHg. (120 is your systolic number, 80 is your diastolic number)
- High blood pressure is when your blood pressure is 140/90 mmHg or greater.
- "Pre-hypertension" is when your blood pressure is greater than 120/ 80 mmHg, but less than 140/90 mmHg. When you have pre-hypertension, you may be at risk for high blood pressure and other health related problems.
- If you have diabetes or kidney problems, your blood pressure should be less than 130/80 mmHg.

What changes can I make in my life if I have high blood pressure?

High blood pressure needs to be controlled. You can change or control some lifestyle habits that will help treat, prevent or delay high blood pressure. These include:

- Healthy eating - choosing a low salt or no salt diet
- Staying physically active
- Keeping or getting to a healthy weight
- Quitting smoking
- Limiting alcoholic drinks to 1-2 a day
- Dealing with stress in a healthy way

- Taking your high blood pressure medicine as prescribed
- Keeping all appointments with your doctor
- Know your blood pressure numbers. Write them down and keep a record.
- Ask your doctor about a home blood pressure monitoring kit and what you need to do to help lower your blood pressure.

Heart Disease

There are many types of heart and blood vessel diseases. Each year more than 870,000 people die from them. Carrying a diagnosis of diabetes increases your chance of having a heart attack or stroke tremendously. Here are some key steps you can take:

- Don't smoke and avoid other people's tobacco smoke.
- Be physically active.
- Keep your weight under control.
- Get regular medical checkups.
- Eat a healthy diet low in saturated fat, cholesterol and salt.
- Control your blood sugar if you have diabetes.

Hardening of the arteries, or atherosclerosis, is when the inner walls of arteries become narrower due to a buildup of plaque. This limits the flow of blood to the heart and brain. Sometimes this plaque can break open. When this happens, a blood clot forms and blocks the artery. This can cause heart attacks and strokes.

Heart attacks occur when the blood flow to a part of the heart is blocked, usually by a blood clot. If this clot cuts off the blood flow completely, the part of the heart muscle supplied by that artery begins to die. Here are some of the signs that can mean a heart attack is happening:

- Uncomfortable pressure, squeezing, fullness or pain in the center of your chest. It lasts more than a few minutes, or goes away and comes back.
- Pain or discomfort in one or both arms.
- Shortness of breath with or without chest discomfort.
- Other signs such as breaking out in a cold sweat, nausea or lightheadedness.

If you have one or more of these signs, don't wait more than 5 minutes before calling for help. Call 9-1-1. Get to a hospital right away.

Strokes

Strokes and Transient Ischemic Attacks (TIA - "mini-stroke") happen when a blood vessel that feeds the brain gets clogged or bursts. Then that part of the brain can't work and neither can the part of the body it controls. Major causes of stroke include:

- High blood pressure
- Smoking
- Diabetes
- High cholesterol
- Heart disease
- Atrial fibrillation (Abnormal heart rhythm)

There are some imaging tests that may be used to help determine your risk for possible heart attack or stroke: (Please refer to Chapter 3)

- Stroke/carotid artery ultrasound – a test used to measure blockages in the arteries that supply the brain. This test is recommended for people with risk factors for vascular disease like hypertension

Call 9-1-1 to get help fast if you have any of these warning signs of stroke and TIA:

- Sudden numbness or weakness of the face, arm or leg, especially on one side of the body.
- Sudden confusion, trouble speaking or understanding.
- Sudden trouble seeing in one or both eyes.
- Sudden trouble walking, dizziness, loss of balance or coordination.
- Sudden, severe headache with no known cause.

16 | Diabetes and Tobacco

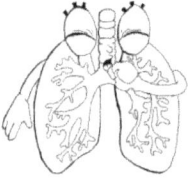

"Smoking is hateful to the nose, harmful to the brain and dangerous to the lungs."

King James I (1566-1625)

By now, you are well aware that smoking damages your heart and lungs. Even today, tobacco use is the second cause of death globally (after high blood pressure) and is currently responsible for killing one in ten adults worldwide. Tobacco use increases the risk of micro and macrovascular complications of diabetes. This increased vascular risk attributable to smoking returns to baseline soon after cessation of tobacco use emphasizing the importance of intervention.

If you smoke, quitting is the number one thing that you can do to improve your standard of living, more than diet, exercise, medications, or rehab.

What does smoking do to my Body?

- Smoking not only damages your lungs, but also many other vital parts of your body. It causes bad breath, accelerates skin aging, reduces fertility, and causes impotence. It also results in increased blood sugar and makes diabetes worse

How do I know how addicted I am to cigarettes?

Most people who smoke will be able to tell you how many cigarettes they smoke in a day. They may also be able to tell how addicted they are to smoking. Below you will find a simple scale to assess how addicted you are to cigarettes.

Fagerström Nicotine Dependence Scale

	0	1	2	3
How soon after you wake up do you smoke your first cigarette?	After 60 minutes	31-60 Minutes	6-30 Minutes	Within 5 minutes
Do you find it difficult to refrain from smoking in places where it is forbidden, e.g., in church, at the library, cinema, etc?	No	Yes		
Which cigarette would you hate most to give up?	All Others	First one in the morning		
How many cigarettes/day do you smoke?	10 or less	11-20	21-30	31 or more
Do you smoke more frequently during the first hours of waking than during the rest of the day?	No	Yes		
Do you smoke if you are so ill that you are in bed most of the day?	No	Yes		

Heatherton TF, Kozlowski LT, Frecker RC, Fagerström KO. The Fagerström Test for Nicotine Dependence: a revision of the Fagerström Tolerance Questionnaire. Br J Addict. 1991 Sep;86(9):1119-27.

Scoring of Fagerström Nicotine Dependency Scale

Three yes/no items are scored 0 (no) and 1 (yes). The 3 multiple-choice items are scored from 0 to 3.

0-2	Very Low Dependence
3-4	Low Dependence
5	Moderate Dependence
6-7	High Dependence
8-10	Very High Dependence

Why is nicotine so addictive? Immediate effects

- Sends nicotine to your brain within 10 seconds.
- Makes you feel more calm and alert.
- You enjoy the feeling so you continue to smoke.

Just one puff... Long-term effects

- The chemical structure of your brain changes - it wants more nicotine to have the same effect.
- You become addicted – you associate your daily routine with cravings to make sure you get a steady flow of nicotine.
- The role of cigarettes becomes important in your life as the brain consistently looks for a nicotine fix.

Benefits of Quitting

Levels of toxic substances that are carried to your lungs in cigarette smoke will drop to those of a non-smoker within a few days, which means your lungs will be able to take in more oxygen, which will make it easier for you to breathe.

After a few weeks your airways will become less inflamed, which means you will cough less, produce less phlegm, and you will gradually find it easier to exercise. It will also improve your blood sugars and the control her diabetes will become much easier.

Once you quit smoking by 12 -18 months most of the increased risk has disappeared and by 3-5 years the risk of vascular complications are the same as that of a nonsmoker.

Reduce your chance of developing lung cancer. After 15–20 years, the risk of lung cancer is reduced substantially compared with people who continue to smoke.

Setting a Quit Date

No one pretends giving up smoking is easy, but if you have made up your mind to quit, you can succeed. It is important to set a date on which you plan to quit smoking (quit-date) and mentally prepare to achieve you set out goal. Use simple tricks to reduce your urge to smoke and help you quit. Look for triggers and plan to avoid them. Consider nicotine replacement therapy or other pharmacotherapeutic agents (Table 5). If you need information or support please call 1-800 QUITNOW.

How to Prevent Relapses of Smoking

- Remind yourself why you gave up smoking in the first place.
- Move away from the area of smokers.
- Keep busy to distract your mind: daily exercise is a good 'distraction' to promote continued abstinence, while counteracting weight gain.
- Drink plenty of water and take deep breaths.

Some triggers for smoking only reveal themselves after you try to live without cigarettes. Tricks that work for some people may not work for others, so quitting can involve trial and error. Keep going! Ask your doctor or nurse for help. Contact a telephone or internet helpline. The most important thing is to be determined and to persist.

If at first you don't succeed, try again…

Nicotine addiction is very powerful and only 5–10% of 'quit attempts' are successful. Withdrawal symptoms, such as craving, irritability, inability to sleep, mood swings, hunger, and headache that occur when the brain is looking for a new fix of nicotine, are a common reason for relapsing and treatment can help this.

Treatment options

Nicotine replacement products such as gum, patches, inhalers and lozenges can help relieve withdrawal symptoms by delivering small, measured doses of nicotine into your body. Evidence shows that anti-smoking medications can double or even triple your chances of being able to quit. Alternative treatments that doctors recommend for heavy smokers are non-nicotine drugs, such as Buproprion SR (Zyban®) and Varenicline tartrate (Chantix®). They are also effective in relieving the cravings and withdrawal symptoms. The idea of taking a drug to kick a drug habit can make people nervous. Some fear unpleasant side effects, while others fear that one addiction will replace another. But smoking is so dangerous for your health that if you weigh the options, (i.e. taking medication or continuing to smoke), using drugs to help you give up smoking will almost always be safer. (See Table 7)

Electronic Cigarettes

Electronic cigarettes or e-cigarettes are electronic nicotine delivery systems (ENDS) that are meant to simulate and substitute for traditional smoking implements, such as cigarettes or cigars, in their use and/or appearance. It generally utilizes a heating element that vaporizes a liquid. Some release nicotine, while others merely release flavored vapor. It substitutes the hand to mouth ritual that most smokers are used to. The risks and benefits of electronic cigarettes are uncertain but they are prescribed as a smoking cessation device.

Table 7: Smoking Cessation Medications

Medications	Dose	Duration	Adverse Effects
Varenicline	1 mg bid	12 weeks if quit attempt, can be extended another 12 weeks.	Nausea
Bupropion SR (slow release)	150 mg every day for 3 d. then 150 mg BID (begin 1-2 weeks pre-quit)	7-12 weeks, maintenance up to 6 months	Insomnia, dry mouth Caution: history of seizures disorder
Nicotine gum	2 or 4 mg gum	Up to 12 weeks	Mouth sores
Nicotine inhaler	6-16 cartridges/day	Up to 6 months	Irritation of mouth & throat
Nicotine nasal spray	8-40 doses/day	3-6 months	Nasal irritation
Nicotine patch	7 -21 mg patch	2-4 weeks	Local skin irritation, insomnia
Nicotine Lozenges	2 -4 mg lozenge	8 weeks	Mouth sores

Don't mistake pleasure for HAPPINESS

17 | Other Endocrine Conditions

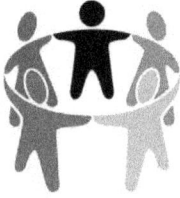

"Helping others is good, Teaching them to help themselves is better."

- George Orwell

Diabetes is considered a disease of the endocrine system as it involves the pancreas which is considered a glandular organ. In this chapter we would like to outline other common endocrine disorders, some of which are commonly seen in diabetes.

Thyroid Disorders

The thyroid gland is located in the neck, just below your larynx (voice box). The thyroid gland produces two thyroid hormones, triiodothyronine (T3) and thyroxine (T4), which regulates the body's metabolic function. Thyroid function is controlled by thyroid-stimulating hormone (TSH), produced in the brain, which tells the thyroid to make T3 and T4.

Hypothyroidism

Hypothyroidism is a term used when you have you have low levels of thyroid hormone. Hypothyroidism is the most common thyroid disorder, it occurs more often in women and tends to be familial. Some symptoms include weight gain, cold intolerance, mental depression, fatigue, dry skin, hair loss and constipation.

These symptoms are not unique to hypothyroidism. A simple blood test can tell whether the symptoms are due to hypothyroidism or some other cause. People with mild hypothyroidism may not have any symptoms at all.

There are many causes of hypothyroidism, but the most common is autoimmune, when the body attacks itself. A condition called Hashimoto's thyroiditis is the most common cause of hypothyroidism. Hypothyroidism can also be caused by radioactive iodine treatment or surgery on the thyroid gland.

Treatment of hypothyroidism is based on thyroid hormone replacement. This is done orally with Levothyroxine as the drug of choice. It is a man-made form of T4 that is identical to the T4 the thyroid naturally makes. Levothyroxine comes in brand-names such as Synthroid® and Levoxyl®. Most people will require thyroid hormone replacement for life. If the brand or dosage needs to be changed, you should have blood tests for TSH done again. Your dose will be adjusted based on your TSH tests.

Hyperthyroidism

Hyperthyroidism is a condition in which the thyroid gland is overactive and too much thyroid hormone is produced. Untreated, this could lead to other health problems involving the heart, bones and liver. Some signs and symptoms of hyperthyroidism may include muscle weakness, heat intolerance, fatigue, weight loss, tremors, irregular heartbeat, diarrhea, as well as other symptoms.

The most common cause of hyperthyroidism is Graves' disease. It occurs when the immune system attacks the thyroid gland, causing it to enlarge and make too much thyroid hormone. Other causes of hyperthyroidism may be a thyroid hormone producing nodule, acute inflammation of the thyroid gland (usually self limiting), and after pregnancy.

How are thyroid disorders diagnosed?

Diagnosis of thyroid disorders relies primarily on blood work and physical examination. Blood tests can measure your levels of thyroid-stimulating hormone (TSH) and thyroid hormone (T4). In hypothyroidism your blood work will show elevated levels of TSH and low levels of T4 and T3 Vice-versa is true in hyperthyroidism. To determine if there is an autoimmune component to your thyroid disorder, blood tests can detect anti-thyroid antibodies that attack the thyroid. Your doctor will also perform a physical examination and may order some other test like an electrocardiogram (EKG) and thyroid ultrasound.

Treatment for hyperthyroidism will depend on its cause, your age and physical condition, and how serious your thyroid problem is. The easiest and most common form of treatment is anti-thyroid medications which reduce the amount of thyroid hormone that your body makes. Examples of these medications are methimazole and propylthiouracil (PTU). Another option is radioactive iodine. This treatment will cure the thyroid problem but leads to hypothyroidism and then thyroid supplementation will have to be initiated. Another option is surgery. Surgical removal of the thyroid gland (thyroidectomy) is a permanent solution, but is now uncommon due to risks to the nearby parathyroids and nerves. Surgery is usually indicated when medications have failed to work or are not an option. Occasionally beta blockers may be prescribed for symptomatic relief. These drugs (such as atenolol) do not lower thyroid hormone levels, but can control many troubling symptoms, especially rapid heart rate, trembling, and anxiety.

Parathyroid Disorders

The parathyroid glands are four pea-sized glands located in your neck inside or slightly behind your thyroid gland. The purpose of the parathyroid glands is to produce parathyroid hormone (PTH) which plays an important role in bone development. PTH helps regulate the level of calcium in your body by having an effect on the bones and kidneys. PTH works in conjunction with phosphorus, which helps your kidneys, muscles and heart work properly and Vitamin D which helps the body absorb calcium.

Hypoparathyroidism

Hypoparathyroidism is the condition in which your body does not make enough PTH. When the level of PTH is diminished the level of calcium in your blood can fall and the levels of phosphorus can rise, which could lead to health problems. It can be caused by surgery of the thyroid, radiation or deficiencies in magnesium. Some symptoms may be muscle spasms, cramps, and/or pain in your legs, feet or face, Weakness, Hair loss, dry hair and skin, and tingling in your fingers, toes, and lips.

If hypoparathyroidism is prolonged it may lead to lead to kidney problems, heart problems, and calcium deposits in the brain. Parathyroid disorders may be diagnosed via simple blood tests to check levels of calcium, phosphorus, magnesium, and PTH.

Treatment for hypoparathyroidism will require you to take calcium and vitamin D supplements to keep your blood calcium levels normal. Depending on the cause of your hypoparathyroidism, you may need to take the supplements for the rest of your life. Your doctor will check your blood levels regularly.

If your blood calcium level becomes extremely low, it can be dangerous for your health. Then you will be given calcium through a vein (IV) and your heart will be checked to make sure it's OK. Once your calcium level is normal, you can go back to taking oral supplements. You might need to follow a diet high in calcium and low in phosphorus. A registered dietitian can help you plan a special diet.

18 | Osteoporosis

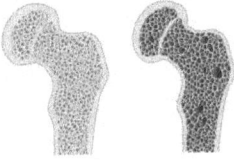

"Nobody travels on the road to success without a puncture or two."

Navjot Singh Sidhu (b. 1963)

Bone is composed of bone cells, collagen, calcium and phosphorus. Bone accrual occurs steadily through childhood and 40%-50% of bone mineral accrual occurs during the teenage years into the early twenties. During this process bone is built, broken down and rebuilt to improve the strength of bone. The majority of this bone accrual is determined by genetics, but factors such as diet and exercise contribute. With aging, the amount of bone that is broken down exceeds the amount of bone that is built and individuals whose bone accrual during the teenage years is sub-optimal are at increased risk for osteoporosis later in life. However, pulmonary patients (both male and female) are often at higher risk for losing bone mass, especially those with more advanced disease.

When bones begin to lose their mass, they are prone to fractures, including compression and fragility fractures. Fractures that occur in the vertebrae (spine), hip and ribs can be particularly problematic. These pathologic fractures lead to decrease of mobility. Fractures in the spine may lead to a hunching effect called kyphosis. Kyphosis restricts the expanding of the lungs which may worsen or exacerbate lung disease.

You should discuss your risk of osteoporosis with your doctor and how to prevent bone loss. This means getting a bone density test, ensuring that you have enough calcium and vitamin D in your diet. Make sure that you are getting rechecked as often as your doctor recommends, especially if you are taking prednisone or other steroids. Prevention of osteoporosis and maintaining healthy bones can be a great asset in your fight against lung disease.

Risk Factors for Osteoporosis:

- Glucocorticoids (e.g. prednisone, etc.) decrease bone formation
- Age related decreased in sex hormones leads to bone loss
- Poor nutrition and malabsorption can lead to deficiencies in vitamins and minerals that are important for the bones (D, K, Zinc, Ca).
- Lack of exercise and decreased weight-bearing activity leads to decreased muscle mass.
- Inflammation can also increase bone loss
- Renal disease can increase bone loss

Individuals with advanced lung disease will require serial DEXA evaluations depending on their bone mineral density (BMD) score. If the DEXA is normal (BMD > T -1) then the DEXA can be repeated in five years (sooner if concerns arise). If the BMD T score is between -1 and -2 the DEXA can be repeated every 2-4 years (again, sooner if concerns arise). A yearly DEXA is recommended for BMD T score of less than -2.

Prevention of poor bone health focuses on overall good nutrition, adequate supplementation of calcium, vitamin D and other vitamins and minerals, regular weight bearing exercise and avoiding excessive glucocorticoid use if possible.

Treatment is indicated for individuals who have a BMD T score of < -2. For individual's whose BMD T-score is between -1 and -2, treatment should be considered if the individual has had what is referred to as a fragility fracture (spine, rib), or if excessive loss has occurred.

Treatment options for osteoporosis in the elderly have expanded over the past few years. Biphosphonates are the mainstay of therapy. These medications prevent bone loss. Zolendronic Acid (delivered intravenously) and oral bisphosphonates increase bone mineral density and appear to decrease fracture risk in adults. Other options for steroid induced osteoporosis, include teriparatide (Forteo®)

In the otherwise healthy population, increasing treatment strategies are becoming available to prevent and treat osteoporosis in the elderly. As individuals with advance lung disease age menopause and senile osteoporosis are additional realities, the role of bone preservation in childhood and early adult years becomes even more relevant.

List of Medications Used for Osteoporosis

Class of Medication	Generic Name	Trade Name®
Natural Supplement	Calcium Vitamin D	Multiple Multiple
Oral Biphosphonares	Alendronate Ibandronate Risedronate	Fosamax Boniva Actonel
IV Biphosphonates	Ibandronate Zoledonic Acid	Boniva Reclast
Monoclonal Antibody	Denosumab	Prolia
Parathyroid Hormone	Teriparatide	Forteo
Selective Estrogen Receptor Modulator (SERM)	Raloxifene	Evista
Hormone Therapy	Estrogen only • Estradiol • Estropipate • Conjugated Estrogens Combination Therapy • Conjugated estrogen & medroxyprogesterone	Estrace Ogen Premarin Prempro
	Calcitonin	Liacalcin, Fortical

"

Your illness does not define you. Your strength and courage does.

"

19 | Diabetes and Social Life

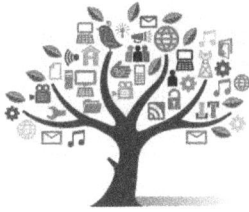

"The biggest disease this day and age is that of people feeling unloved."

Princess Diana (1961-1997)

A diagnosis of diabetes may cause you to feel sad and worried about your future. These feelings may manifest as depression, which can have a detrimental effect on your overall health. Depression is a condition that is caused by a combination of psychological, physical, and in some case genetic factors.

Depression can also make it difficult to take care of yourself and your disease properly. When this feeling sets in, you may also want to stop fighting your disease and miss medications. You may think that it is pointless to exercise, or that they are not able to do enough to make a difference. All this can make living with diabetes worse.

Doctors have known for years that sleep problems are intertwined with mood disorder. Poor sleep (insomnia) is a symptom of depression. Full blown insomnia is more serious than sleep problems that many people occasionally have. To qualify for a diagnosis, people must have endured at least a month of chronic sleep loss that causes problems at work, home or important relationships. Developing insomnia doubles the chances of later on being depressed i.e. the sleep problem precedes the mood disorder (depression).

Cognitive behavior therapy for insomnia may help. It is thought to teach people how to establish a regular wake up time and how to stick to it; how to get out of bed while awake and how to avoid eating, reading, watching television and to eliminating similar activities.

The aim is to restrict time in bed for sleeping only and to curb the idea that sleeping needs effort and to establish that going to bed is for sleeping only.

Depression

The symptoms of depression are commonly described by the acronym SIG-E-CAPS. You must have 2 or more of the following symptoms on most days for at least 2 weeks duration to have a diagnose of depression

- Sleep changes: increase during day or decreased sleep at night
- Interest (loss): of interest in activities that used to interest them
- Guilt (worthless): depressed elderly tend to devalue themselves
- Energy (lack): common presenting symptom (fatigue)
- Cognition/Concentration: reduced cognition &/or difficulty concentrating
- Appetite (wt. loss); usually declined, occasionally increased
- Psychomotor: agitation (anxiety) or retardations (lethargic)
- Suicidal thoughts

Management of Depression

Depression may be managed in many ways. The first step to management is acknowledging the way you feel and actively seeking help. Conservatively it may be managed by talking to someone. This may be a family member, a psychologist, or you may even attend a support group meeting. Depression may also be managed with cognitive behavior therapy (CBT), a form of psychotherapy that trains people to view their feelings in a more positive way and to cope with the stresses of living with a chronic disease. Some people may find the above therapies enough but others may also need to use anti-depressant medications (See Appendix 5). Antidepressant medications work by changing the concentration of neurotransmitters (signaling chemicals) in the brain. These medications take some time to reach their effective levels and may take up to one month before you see results. Eventually, these medications may be able to restore your sense of well-being. More recently it has been shown that physical activity improves mental well-being. Living with advanced lung disease, physical activity may benefit both your mental and physical health.

List of Depression Medications

Type of Medication	Generic Names	Trade Names®
Selective serotonin-reuptake inhibitor (SSRIs)	Fluoxetine Sertraline Paroxetine Citalopram Escitalopram Fluvoxamine	Prozac Zoloft Paxil Celexa Lexapro Luvox
Serotonin-norepinephrine reuptake inhibitor (SNRIs)	Venlafaxine Duloxetine Desvenlafaxine	Effexor Cymbalta Pristiq
Atypical antidepressant	Bupropion Mirtazepine Trazodone	Wellbutrin, Zyban Remeron Desyrel
Tricyclic antidepressant (TCAs)	Amitriptyline Clomipramine Desipramine Doxepine Imipramine Nortriptyline Protriptyline Maprotilin	Elavil Anafranil Norpramin, Sinequan, Adapin Tofranil Aventyl, Pamelor Vivactil, Triptil Ludiomil
Monoamine oxidase inhibitors (MAOs)	Isocarboxazid Phenelzine Tranylcypromine	Marplan Nardil Parnate

Appendix

Useful Contact Information

American Diabetes Association
1701 North Beauregard Street
Alexandria, VA 22311   1-800-DIABETES
http://www.diabetes.org

American Sleep Apnea Association
6856 Eastern Avenue NW Suite 203
Washington, DC 20012   1-888 293-3650
http://www.sleepapnea.org/